Free Me 2 Be Me

MY TURBULENT JOURNEY WITH BREAST CANCER

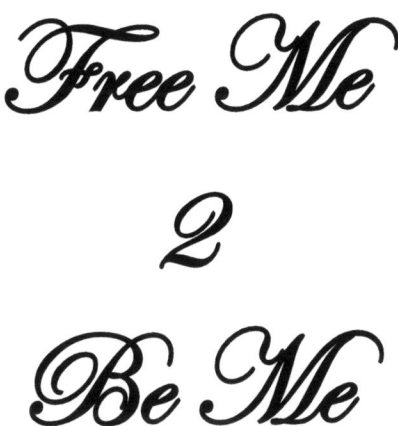

Free Me 2 Be Me

MY TURBULENT JOURNEY WITH BREAST CANCER

Erika Weathers

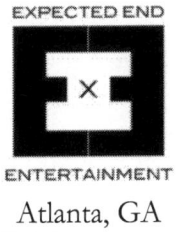

Atlanta, GA

Copyright © 2021 Erika Weathers
Cover Images: Photography by Amelia Design
Author Headshot: Ira Carmichael Photography
Photo Graphics: Richard Watkins

All rights reserved. No part of this book may be reproduced or transmitted in any form or by any means, electronic or mechanical, including photocopy, recording, or by any information storage and retrieval system with the exception of a reviewer who may quote brief passages in a review to be printed in a blog, newspaper or magazine without written permission from the author. Address inquiries to: iamerikaweathers@gmail.com

Published with assistance from Expected End Entertainment
ISBN: 978-1-7371462-2-3

Printed in the United States of America

CONTENTS

	INTRODUCTION	1
1	ANALYZE THIS	5
2	HELLO, IT'S ERIKA WITH A K	21
3	WHAT THE HELL	43
4	LOVE THYSELF	55
5	BACK TO LIFE	71
6	MENTOR, MENTOR WHERE FOR	79
7	PERCEPTION	89
8	IT'S BACK	105
9	TAKE ADVANTAGE OF WHATEVER	113
10	LOOK AT ME NOW	129
	ABOUT THE AUTHOR	141

DEDICATION

To My Mother, Jacqueline Zoldan, who has always been there for me when I needed her most. I Love You, Mommy!

ACKNOWLEDGMENTS

To everyone who has inspired me, challenged me, and even doubted me to write this. THANK YOU! To my family and friends, I pray this book doesn't disappoint you. I pray it heals you in a way that it has helped heal me. I hope you all are as proud of me as I am of myself!

ERIKA WEATHERS

INTRODUCTION

ERIKA WEATHERS

Free Me 2 Be Me is a book about freeing yourself, forgiving yourself, and loving yourself. It's never too late to make changes in your life and to set new goals because anything is possible if you work hard for it. As a breast cancer survivor, losing a breast should be the least of my worries. I'm still here. I'm still living. Instead of feeling sorry for ourselves, we need to continue to live in all our glory...striving and thriving.

I am blessed to still be here. Many breast cancer patients haven't been so lucky. We really need to start looking at life differently. It may have taken me 40 years to get here, but hopefully you'll follow your path in your 20s, 30s, 40s, 50s or 60s. Whatever your age, find the passion in your life that will make you happy and remove the toxins, bad relationships, bad habits and bad behaviors. Start seeing the miracles that will happen in your life. Don't be afraid to leave that job, or relationship, or city. Take a chance to follow your passion in life. If it takes a pandemic to light a fire under you, so be it. It's time to make a change for the better.

The things that I accomplished in less than a year amaze me. It lets me know when I set a goal and put my all into it, it can be done. I finished my first book. I am now a notary, a real estate agent, still a student completing my AA in criminal justice, and the possibility of obtaining my bachelors, a new flight attendant with an old company, and still an aspiring actress waiting to book that next gig. We have to remember that being proud of ourselves can be more important than making others proud of us. Believe that you are enough! Be a risk taker, dare yourself, and remember... you can accomplish anything you put your mind, body and your soul into.

FREE ME 2 BE ME

I wanted to write this book to share my story of that little mixed girl who wanted to be white and who is now so proud to be a black woman. You should never be ashamed of who you are and where you come from. Take advantage of any opportunity to educate yourself because it will open doors for you to maneuver your way through this world. Never second guess yourself and if you need some help, ask for it. We all make mistakes but those mistakes can be turned into miracles.

ERIKA WEATHERS

CHAPTER ONE

ANALYZE THIS

OBSESSION: a persistent disturbing preoccupation with an often unreasonable idea or feeling.
Infatuation, fetish, fixation, passion…

ERIKA WEATHERS

I analyze everything, think it over in my mind and wish I would have said this or asked that. I think about what I could have done to make it better. I find it hard to be in the moment... to live and let live... to not overthink or obsess about everything, instead of just doing it! My mantra was always, "Don't sweat the small stuff" and I still believe that today. I always try to let things slide off my back and keep it moving.

I recently met a man on the plane who was an author. He gave me a copy of his new book, "The Little Things: Why You Really Should Sweat the Small Stuff". He made me think about my motto and told me that if you keep letting those small things roll off your back, they could turn into bigger issues that will eventually be harder to deal with. I was like, "You got something there." I guess I have to find a new favorite motto.

We all want to do better, we just don't know how to get there, or how to follow through. How many people start a project, a mission, or set a goal but never complete it? Why? What is the mental block? Is it that we don't know how to get there by ourselves or don't want to ask for help? For example, I have been wanting to write this book for a long time, but I could never get the words from my notebook to my computer. I was coming up on a milestone and started branding myself on Instagram. I was trying to get more followers that would help me sell my book and also help with my acting. In this new world, you could get a gig for having thousands and millions of followers.

I hired a woman to help get me going. She gave me great ideas, helped me with my posts, mission statement, and a photo shoot. From these works, I was getting a lot more followers but they seemed to be from other parts of the world, not really in the USA. We weren't buying them but it was an algorithm that would boost who could see your posts and what hashtags to use. Every day, I either posted inspirational photos or I wrote my own quote on photos of myself from the photo shoot. It was a lot. I did it for a couple months but it just got so overwhelming. So I stopped. I still post but not every day. It's so crazy how for 3 months I was posting something inspirational or positive or a picture of myself, and I got the most likes of pictures of myself. They were all pretty sexy and cute. Some were professionally done, but most were from my girlfriend Eloise. She would come over and snap away. We got some great shots. My acting friends would be like, "Are you trying to be a model, too?" It's crazy how people get judgmental or have an opinion about my posts but then don't even like them. So many "lookie loos". Most of the likes are from the ladies. You know the guys are looking, but they only like your pictures here and there.

My target date was going to be my 10-year cancer-free anniversary but I didn't make it. That's when the writer's block kicked in and I got stuck. I had a lot going on. I was still flying, back in school getting my associates degree in art, attending my acting classes, trying to brand myself, and write this book all on a deadline. I put too much pressure on myself. When your road map isn't outlined perfectly, you eventually end up of course. When I didn't complete the book for my 10-year anniversary, my focus on the book stopped. It took me another three years to get it done.

Nothing is perfect. When we get off course, we must regroup and get back on track. That's what I'm doing... getting it done!

I'm a glass half-full type of girl in almost every aspect of my life. I try to see the best in people and give them the benefit of the doubt. I trust and trust some more, even when I can see the truth staring me right in my face. So when I had to come face-to-face and battle cancer twice, I did it punching and kicking the whole way. I believed that I would overcome it, do whatever I needed to do to kill it, conquer it and destroy it so that there wasn't a third time! I needed and wanted to get my life back on track. I was in my early 30s when I was first diagnosed and my late 30s when it came back. I was still single with no kids. I still had the opportunity to get pregnant, but with no real prospects, my window was getting smaller. I wanted to be married again and have a baby. I'm a strong believer that what you put into the universe will come back to you tenfold. I believe that positivity will always overcome negative energy, pessimistic people and the nastiness in the world.

It can be a hard mindset to develop because I have witnessed the good and the bad and the ugliness of relationships, friendships, and family. Letting go, forgiving, and moving on can the best thing you can do for your mind, body and soul. I realize that I can't obsess about every little thing and that I'm not always the problem. At the end of the day, when someone tells you it's not you, just believe that. They may just be having a bad day or there might be a bigger issue involved and you're just the scapegoat. It is what it is! If it can't be fixed or if it's not worthy of your time, let it go and move on. I now realize you have to forgive for real for real. You cannot let it fester because it will only do harm to you. Like the song from the movie "Frozen" says... Let it go!

Yes, I still have my moments. It's so easy to be negative. People thrive on negativity, secretly hoping things don't work out for you. They make excuses to stay away from you when you need them or simply don't show up. I've had to learn to spend time with the right people, make happiness a daily priority, practice what I preach, use the power of self-reflection, and let go of self-limiting behaviors. Otherwise, I will be a carrier of that negativity.

Believe me, I know that I am a work in progress. I can be a real bitch when I'm pushed. I even have a great resting bitch face and I'm told that I'm not very approachable at first glance. I'm told that I carry myself as a sexy, confident woman with a striking presence that has a walk that could stop traffic and a smile that can light up a room... that is, when I DO smile. When you get to know the real Erika, you will see that I am as beautiful on the inside as I am on the outside. But I will let you all be the judge of that. Take the time to get to know me before you judge me and I will do the same. So, what does all this mean? We all judge each other for one reason or another. That first impression, that feeling, that idea or opinion, is all based on little evidence. It's all based on everything going on outside of us. We haven't even opened our mouths yet and we are already being judged or perceived a certain way. But that is what we do. We make up our minds and make judgements on people we don't even know. We already hate them, envy them, love them, and without admitting it, want to be them.

Everyone you encounter enters your life for a reason, a season or a lifetime. Sometimes, that person is a stranger who may enter your life in a way that touches you in that moment, giving you something you needed to hear. You may wonder, "What the heck was that?" It all usually makes sense at some point in our lives. We just have to listen, interpret and take it in. There are those boyfriends who have served their purpose but you then realize they were what you needed at the time. Then there's that girlfriend who helped you realize this is not how I want to live my life anymore. There's that family member who you try to help but realize they don't even want it, the relationship is just too stressful, and/or really not worth all the crap that comes with it.

I have two best girlfriends in my life who I have known since we were in grade school. I've known one of them since fifth grade. Pam has always been my biggest cheerleader. We were cheerleaders in grade school together. She has always had my back and will tell me the truth... good or bad. I found a letter she sent me when I was living with my dad and stepmother for a semester back in 1983, before I went back to live with my mom over some drama with my older brother. It was so funny, like Pam didn't think my parents would open it. It said, "For Erika's Eyes Only". She made a wonderful toast at my 50th birthday dinner.

We moved around a lot when I was growing up. After my mom divorced for the second time, we moved out to Scotchtown. Pam and I were cheerleaders and we didn't live too far from each other. It was a great neighborhood. Jennifer, another good friend, lived right up the street from Pam. I met Kathy and her sister Jenny (who were a year younger than us) in junior high school. We played softball together. Their family invited me into their home my senior year when my mom didn't get a place big enough for me to have my own bedroom. I could have stayed on the couch living with my mom, but Kathy offered her home, her room and her bed to share with me. So, I took her up on the offer. The house was full. Her mom and dad, her grandma, her sister and little brother, a cat and dog, plus me. They were all so welcoming... such a loving family. We don't talk every day but we all know that we are just a call or text away. We try to get together several times a year for drinks, dinner, a Broadway show, our 20th class reunion, or a weekend to just catch up. We went to the beach in Destin for our 40th birthdays, to The Finger Lakes in New York was a fascinating and quaint place and a late 50s celebration in Hawaii in Kona in 2020. One of the best perks of my job is the free travel to visit family and friends or having a great overnight in a city where I can meet up with them.

I went with Pam and Kathy to my first Broadway show (*The Color Purple*) in New York City. It was so great. I came up another time just for the day to see Denzel Washington in the *Iceman Cometh*. One of the perks of being an aspiring actress is I can really appreciate what goes into the work. I know it will be difficult but I'm going to try and book a play this year. I know when I did a showcase with my acting class I had so much fun and our scene was one of the funniest of the night. I know it will take my acting skills to another level along with building my confidence.

Our trip to Destin, Florida, was so fabulous. It was the six of us... Pam, Kathy, my cousin Dawn, Jenny and Sue. We rented a condo on the beach. The white sand was probably the best, most perfect sand ever. Bermuda is a close second. Their beaches are beautiful as well. We took a picture of the four of us (Jenny, Kathy, Pam and I) in our bathing suits. I tried to replicate the picture in Hawaii but the girls weren't having it! We did one fully clothed. Actually, Pam and I wore bathing suits. We are the two who haven't had kids and workout on a regular basis. Pam works out more than I do, but I'm working on it. The Finger Lakes in Cornell, NY, was a fascinating quaint place. We stayed at an Airbnb right on the lake. The host had wine and vegetables from their garden waiting for us. We went wine tasting and made blown glass figures. It's so funny the hidden treasures you can find in the state you grew up in once you explore it. The state of New York is so big and beautiful. It consists of way more than just New York City. Whenever I tell someone I'm from New York they say, "What borough?", and I say, "I'm from upstate, about an hour north of the city." Their response is, "Oh, you're not from New York." I give them that look like, "Really? Get yourself out of the city and explore the whole state of New York."

I still haven't actually been to Niagara Falls. I have only flown over it, landing and taking off from Toronto which is also beautiful. It's on my bucket list this year or when I get back to traveling. The girls and I are all so different from one another. But what keeps us together is the bond we developed when we were just kids. I know those girls will always be there for me no matter what. They won't judge me, they just accept me for me. Dawn has been in my life pretty much since day one. My father and her mother are brother and sister. We were born the same year, 1969. My birthday is in August and hers is in October, a couple days after my mother's. She really has been by my side, at family reunions reminding me who everyone was, in school when I got in trouble with other kids, teaching me how to fight, or just sticking up for me. We didn't always hang out in the same crowd but we have always been there for each other day or night, good and bad times. She really is more like my sister than a cousin. Shit, I barely talk to my older sister, and my stepsister is in California and I only see her maybe once a year. We only talk a handful of times throughout the year.

Dawn had told me that she used to put me on a pedestal, thinking I had everything she desired until she actually saw that I was just like her. She thought I was the beautiful one, the light skin one, the one who was always favored. She told me she had never received flowers from a man. I couldn't imagine that because that is what I would expect from a man in my life. I love fresh flowers. I would buy them for myself if I was home on a regular basis. It's the small stuff that really does matter. Sometimes, it takes expressing yourself to others so they know what you want and need. I almost sent my cousin flowers but didn't want to seem patronizing. I knew it would still be welcomed and put a smile on her face. Once I felt what others felt, it made me realize that I was given so many blessings from God and I wasn't taking advantage of them. I was using them to get ahead but still blaming someone else for what was wrong with me. It's funny you have to hear someone else's story so you can edit yours and appreciate the things you take for granted, as well as be accepting of things that you deserve. Let the edits begin. Start realizing that your story isn't so bad; it just needs to be tweaked. You are all deserving of the good life (whatever it means to you), even if it is that fake Gucci or Louis.

But I still say, always try to get the real thing, even if it's just the one bag or wallet. I think you will appreciate it even more. Always value yourself and put yourself on a pedestal. Strive for greatness because if you don't look out for yourself, how can you expect others to do it for you? I know I will continue to do that because I deserve it!

I have thought about how I think my cancer started mutating and developing into my breast cancer. I know stress is a big factor. I have experienced stress pretty much my whole life. From my parents divorcing while I was young, to our family being split up, to not growing up with my siblings (especially my twin brother), to keeping secrets about my mom and my older brother, to my father not giving me the love that I needed, to having a difficult relationship with my stepmother. I've been stressed. I know a lot of kids go through divorce, so that's not new. But it's how the parents handle it. My mother and father had two different households after my mom remarried and was introduced to drugs and alcohol. That changed her. So when she got divorced again, she stayed single and continued using drugs and alcohol. She really wasn't there for me. My father also remarried. He was a very strict disciplinarian. It was "his" way or the highway. I always felt like they had somebody watching me to report back to them. He would always know something. It wasn't a comfortable relationship.

I remember developing this skin rash when I was in grade school. It was on my legs, my back, my stomach and some on my forehead. I had to wear a long bang to try and cover it. It was disgusting. It was multiple small scaly, pink or red spots. I had to try and hide it so no one knew what I looked like. It lasted almost six month. It was so bad that it left permanent scars on my legs. It's called pityriasis rosea virus, also known as the Christmas tree virus because the patches are usually oval shaped and often form a pattern on the back that resembles a Christmas tree. I kept so much stuff inside that I guess it had to find other ways to get out. It never came back, thank God, but I do have eczema. It flares up seasonally, but I have dealt with that my whole life.

I was always trying to be someone else, instead of who I was meant to be. I have to start where it all pretty much began because we begin developing who we are at such a young age because of the influences of people around us. We learn behaviors from our parents and siblings, schoolmates and teachers. I felt that I wasn't enough at such a young age. You can see it in my actions and in my choices as I was growing up and becoming an adult. These situations influence who we

FREE ME 2 BE ME

become as adults. They contribute to good and bad behaviors. The way we treat our bodies, our heart, and the lack of self-respect we have, all play a role in who we become and how we treat others. It all makes a difference in our development.

The environment is also a big factor. Toxins and pollutants are culprits. For a period of time, we lived by a perfume factory called Polak's and we smelled those toxic chemicals on a daily basis. My sense of smell was always strong and I remember breathing in the candy-like smell. To this day, I can only wear perfume on special occasions and if I'm around someone with a musky smell or the perfume your grandmother wore, I can't stay around them for long.

I smoked cigarettes, smoked weed, and drank alcohol. We used to do lots of shots. One time, one of my friends went to Linden block. It was a known area in town to get drugs. She went to buy all of us a hit of acid. I had never done it before so I was like, "Ok." I was a follower. I didn't have anything better to do. I didn't even think of the consequences. I don't think I ever thought about consequences. I would just do things. That night, only one of my friends didn't take the acid. She got there late so someone else got hers. Thank God because she ended up taking care of me that night. I had a really bad trip. I thought I was dead. It was like I was in a cartoon and people were yelling peer pressure things at me. Their heads were in a bubble circle around my head and I was just looking back and forth listening. The voices were talking so fast that they were starting to overlay each other and turning into just loud noise. My head was going from side to side, trying to figure out what the hell was going on. I couldn't make it stop. I felt like I was going crazy. I thought I was dead and the whole time my girlfriend said she just stood there holding me while I was shaking. She was so scared and so glad she didn't take one. I was the only one that had a really bad trip. After that episode, I didn't feel the same for a while, if I drank alcohol or smoked weed. I would feel like I was tripping again. I still had side effects, feeling like the acid was still in my system and it was probably turning psychological. I felt like it was playing with my mind. I was paranoid thinking that I would never be the same again. I didn't like the way I felt. I stopped doing everything. No drugs. No alcohol. I was scared. I didn't really tell anyone about it. I just dealt with it myself like I did with most things in my life. That feeling eventually went away and I was back to my partying ways.

From then on, I only did weed and alcohol. I never tried coke. I used to see my mom use it and I didn't like the way she acted. In addition, sniffing something didn't seem appealing or look like fun to me. They would snort it up one nostril, make this face, shake their heads, and then smile while waiting for it to hit. Some would then take the leftover powder and run it across their teeth. I'm glad I never got into it because several of my friends really liked it, especially my mom. It's an addictive drug. A lot of my friends did it but I would just pass. We really were a bunch of drugged up, alcohol drinking teenagers that never had a problem getting anything we wanted. It still amazes me.

I have been a flight attendant for over 20 years and there have been studies that have been going on for years regarding cancer developing from the radiation that we encounter everyday being in the air. The fumes we ingested from the jet fuel that contain carcinogen. There is no real documentation but a lot of flight attendants have the disease. There are so many culprits that cause cancer, like sugar, high fructose syrup, and carcinogens of BBQ from the charred meat.

FREE ME 2 BE ME

I also think never having kids also fueled my cancer growth, with estrogen always continuing to pump in my body. I first had my period at the age of 12, which is considered on the younger side. Also, the use of birth control and the added hormones could be a contributing factor. I am also a twin so maybe that played a factor, too. We didn't share the same egg. We had two sets of egg and sperm fertilized by its own sperm cell and we only share about 50% of our DNA. But who really knows, we all have cancer cells in our body. Some of the cells mutate into cancer and some don't. We probably will never know why anyone develops cancer. It's a big moneymaker, so we probably never will! They will just continue to keep coming up with new and improved treatment plans, costly drugs and better therapies. With all the money that has gone into research over the years, what have they really learned? What have they shared about why someone develops a particular cancer? Have they offered any new information that could help to prevent the spread of the disease or a test that can be taken to let you know that your cells are mutating so you could catch it early? If there was a test, most people probably couldn't even afford it. Just imagine if you had no insurance. You really would be shit out of luck. You wouldn't even go to the doctor, so it could just be growing in your body with no early detection. Then, by the time you do find it, it could be Stage 3 or even worse... terminal. It's just crazy. It just makes me mad!! That's why I believe everyone should have affordable healthcare and get regular checkups to be accountable for yourself and your wellbeing.

I just saw a story on the news about a home test that you could take to see if you had the brca1 or brca2 gene. This lady had a positive result and had her breast and ovaries taken out. The test didn't give a 100% chance that she would get cancer but she was being proactive. She may have gotten cancer but she also could have never gotten cancer. I don't think I could have just removed everything. I would get a second, maybe third, opinion so I could make an informed decision. But everyone is on their own journey and must do what is best for them. People also believe that if they have a double mastectomy that they wouldn't get cancer which is not always true. Being proactive in this way isn't always the best way to go but if it makes you feel better, then go for it. Just be sure to get a second opinion and know all the factors that go along with your decision. Being your own advocate is one of the best things you can do for yourself.

1. Do you see things in life as half-full or half-empty? Why?

_____
_____
_____

2. Do you try to start your day with a positive daily ritual? If so, what is it?

_____
_____
_____

3. Do you tend to hold things in or do you freely speak your mind? Why?

_____
_____
_____

4. Did you have a good childhood? What is your fondest memory?

_____
_____
_____

FREE ME 2 BE ME

5. Is there anything you wished you did differently growing up? Give an example:

_____
_____
_____

> *"I have encountered many defeats, but I won't be defeated. Whenever I doubt myself, I remember how far I have come and I know good things are going to happen! Soon very soon."*

ERIKA WEATHERS

CHAPTER TWO

HELLO, IT'S ERIKA WITH A K

Sex: Sexually motivated phenomena or behavior, copulation, fornication

ERIKA WEATHERS

It all started back in the summer of 1969. I always think of that Bryan Adams song when I say that. Two bouncing babies: one little girl wrapped in pink and one little boy wrapped in blue. Both were about six ounces and some change, arriving about 12:40 p.m. They were about six mins apart, coming in as babies number 3 and 4 to the Weathers Clan. I have an older sister who is six years older, and an older brother four years older. Our parents had been together on and off for at least 10 years until finally divorcing. My father remarried and is still married. From that union, I now have a stepbrother and stepsister. My mom had remarried as well, but divorced again and remains single.

My stepfather, who was white, lived in a very prominent part of town called Presidential Heights. Maybe this is where I realized that this was the kind of lifestyle I wanted. I knew that I didn't want to end up in the projects like my mom's mother, my nanny or like my aunt or cousins. I guess at a young age I still felt like I was better than that, that I would never want to live in the projects and I still carry myself that way. My sister, on the other hand, liked the projects. She was the one who looked out for us. She was the tough one, a tomboy, the one who would beat your ass in a minute. She was rougher around the edges and liked the thugs that were in and out of jail. I was also a tomboy, but also very girly. I have never been in a fight. Well, I was almost in one when I was in junior high school, but it never happened because I would have been kicked off my softball team. It's so funny my cousin was training me to fight. It was like the whole school knew it was going down. Word got around and my coach put a stop to it. Thank God because I didn't want to fight. I was scared shitless.

I got a glimpse of living like the rich, a glimpse of living like the poor, and a glimpse of everything in between. I knew where I wanted to be, but at that age I didn't have a clue how to get there. I loved my stepfather, but he is the one who had introduced my mom to drugs. When she met him, all the kids had lived with my father. It was a lot for him and my stepmother. Soon, my dad was sick with kidney stones and ended up bringing my brother and I to town to live with my mom and stepfather. That was all short lived. My mom and stepfather divorced not long after that.

I remember our neighbors at the time. I looked up to them because one was a doctor and the other a stewardess. We call them flight attendants now. He used to get a car service to drive her into the city for work. It was about an hour drive to LaGuardia Airport or JFK Airport. I thought it was so glamorous. They also had two adorable kids - a boy named Tyler and girl named Logan, who had red hair. She was so sweet. I loved her name and would one day hope to name my daughter the same. Their lives just seemed so perfect to me. It was just another glimpse of what I could only hope for. We don't really know how impressionable we are at such a young age. Little things stay with us over time that we strive for, not realizing from where they originated. I believe everything goes back to our childhoods and shape who we become, including how our parents raised us or didn't raise us, and the love we receive or the lack of love we receive. Some try to do better with their kids, some make excuses as to why it will be the same old same old because they don't know how to do better.

My mother was half Italian, white and whatever else she was mixed with. She never knew her father; she only had pictures. All her siblings had different fathers. Yes, my nanny was a rolling stone out there and never married. My mom, being the oldest, took most of the abuse from my nanny. It wasn't a great relationship. It had its moments, but my mom didn't get the love and nurturing she needed so she didn't really know how to give it to her own children. My mom never graduated from high school because my nanny had kicked her out and she went to work as a seamstress for little pay. She was also going to beauty school then working in retail before becoming a bartender and dealing drugs to survive as a single parent. She was born in Middletown and has lived there her whole life.

My dad, a black man born in South Carolina, came north in his late teens without graduating from high school. He lived with his sister for a while. He started working in the factory, but also knew construction, spackling, and making furniture. He had his own business for a while because he could pretty much fix anything. He retired from the state working as a corrections officer.

We lived in Orange County, New York, where it was prominently white. My stepmother was white and her kids were white and Jewish. We had all been in each other's lives at a young age. My stepsister was the same age as my twin and I, so we always had a good relationship, and still do. I have a better relationship with her than my older sister. All the kids had gotten separated. My older brother and I lived with my mom in town and my twin and older sister lived with my dad. Both my stepbrother and sister ended up living with their mom and my dad up on the mountain. I always wondered why they split me and my twin up. They would say that my brother was sickly with asthma and wanted to stay with my dad and I wanted to stay with my mom. They also told me I was the bossy one and I would try to do everything before he did it and they didn't think that was good. They said that we needed to be separated at school. I'm still a

FREE ME 2 BE ME

bossy bitch but that's just the Leo in me. I would see my other siblings on some weekends, but it wasn't the same as living together. My brother and I never had that great bond like most twins have. Even with living with my older brother, we didn't have a close bond. He was four years older than me, so when I got into high school he graduated and was getting ready to enter the Air Force. It was like I was an only child when I went into high school. I was a loner. I spent a lot of time by myself because my mom worked at night. I pretty much had to take care of myself, do my homework, have dinner and get ready for the next day. I had so much freedom. No wonder I was looking for attention whenever I got bored.

I didn't have a plan, but I knew New York would not be my future. We lived in the suburbs. We had cows walking in the pasture. It was a nice place to grow up but too slow and too cold in the winter. I did have a job. I first started working at Wendy's then Baskin Robbins, Sears and Mandee's over the years.

As soon as I graduated from high school, I was on a plane to San Diego California. I was running and not looking back. I didn't really know my sister very well; she was in the navy, married with two kids. She was doing very well. We got along well. I really appreciated her affording me a place to stay until I could figure out what to do with my life. I was like a hermit for a while I didn't know anyone. I helped take care of my nephew and niece. They were the cutest babies. Branden looked like a Michelin baby and Brittany a Tweety Bird. I shared a room with my niece until I could get a job, a car and save some money to get my own apartment. I got a telemarketing job, which was horrible. I found another job with a window company doing telemarketing and worked my way to office manager dealing with the sales guy. I was making pretty good money. I took the bus to and from work until I could get a car. I needed to get my driver's license because in New York I just had a permit due to not owning a car. I used to drive Kathy's big old boat and the Mazda. I saved up enough money to buy a Mitsubishi Precis. It was a stick shift and my first brand new car. My brother-in-law taught me how to drive it. I hung out with my sister on base with her at some of the clubs that were for 18 and older and met some guys. But I didn't really make any friends. My sister had cookouts and the neighbor and friends came by. I dated a couple white guy from work but nothing special until I met Reggie Murrell, one of my brother-in-law's friends. I was about 19 and he was about 27 with a son and newly divorced. He never came on to me like all the other guys that used to hang around so I kind of migrated to him. He helped me get home one night. We ended up talking and then I kissed him. At least that's the story that *he* would tell.

Reggie was a sweet guy. He cared for and loved me. He was my first "real" black boyfriend. He was very dark skinned, and you know the old saying... "Once you go black you never go back." And I haven't. Not to say that I wouldn't date a white guy again, but it just hasn't happened. I haven't been attracted to one. It's funny... I'm so much more pro black then when I was a kid. I look at interracial couples and think that it's still too much work. You get the side eye from people even today.

My sister's marriage was starting to show signs that things weren't going in the right direction. Of course, I was blamed for getting her out of the house and getting her back into shape after having the babies. But I didn't have anything to do with it. They both had their own problems, and I don't know who started cheating first. They soon separated and then divorced.

FREE ME 2 BE ME

My sister left the navy and moved back to New York with the kids. I stayed in California and got my own place until Reggie and I eventually got a place together. We had a good relationship. He treated me nicely and made me feel special. We had a good time together and he really loved me. He did have a temper and when he was mad everyone knew it. I was young, just growing into a young lady. My body was just fully developing, and I was still exploring the world, trying to figure out who I was or who I could be. Reggie was also in the navy and had to leave on a westpac for six months. I thought that would be ok, but six months was a long time and I got bored. He had asked me to get married several times and I would always say, "No. Not yet, but soon." I did love him but I wasn't in love with him. It was like he was my security blanket and maybe if he never left me, we would have been ok. Maybe I would have fallen in love with him. That was my first real relationship. I don't think I even really knew what love was or how I was supposed to feel, but I knew I was missing something. Otherwise, I would have married him.

I went back to school to get my certificate to become a travel agent and continued to take classes at the junior college. I started working as a cocktail waitress at a strip club called Pure Platinum. I had to wear this cute tuxedo top that went around our necks with the back out, a purple bow tie and cummerbund, and a G-string with nude opaque tights. So, it appeared as my butt was out. It was really good money. I also started modeling and doing some swimsuit editions for a local TV station, some local commercials, some featured extra work on the TV show Silk Stalkings, and some print work for an athletic company. I lived in San Diego, just two hours from LA but I was never one of those girls that could just pack up and move to LA with stars in my eyes, like I was going to be the next big star. I always had to have a steady job to be able to pay my bills.

I made a good friend working at the club and we started going out to nightclubs having a great time. I got hit on at the strip club and most nights made more money than most of the dancers. I ended up meeting an NFL football player named Nate, who played for the San Diego Chargers (now Los Angeles Chargers) at this club called Smokey's. We had so much fun. We started hanging out even though he knew I had a boyfriend. He also had a girlfriend who lived in LA, so it worked for a while. When Reggie came back, I told him I had cheated on him, but he forgave me. I couldn't break up with him because I had hurt him. He still wanted to be with me. He was willing to forgive me and move on. So, we got back into our relationship. It was ok, but Nate was always on my mind. I would run into him at the gas station sometimes. It was crazy because he only lived down the street from me, but I didn't go back to him because he still had his girlfriend. I was trying to make things work with Reggie because he really was a good guy. Well, when Reggie left me again on another westpac, I ended up getting back with Nate. He broke up with his girlfriend and before my boyfriend came back, I broke up with him in a letter. I had to do it before he got back so he couldn't talk me out of it like he did the last time. I know it was horrible, but I should have never stayed with him after cheating on him the first time. When I am fully committed in a relationship, I don't cheat. That's why I told him, figuring he would break up with me, but he didn't.

Reggie was so hurt that we got into a big fight. It was horrible. I felt so bad, but I had to be truthful this time. We went our separate ways.

I hadn't heard from Reggie for a long time until he found me on

FREE ME 2 BE ME

Facebook years later. That's one good thing about Facebook... you can find people from your past, if they are into social media. He would say hi and ask how I was doing from time to time. I finally asked him why he forgave me the first time and why he would have forgiven me a second time for cheating on him. He told me the door was still open for a very long time and that he never truly got over me. He loved me so much that he felt a connection with me. Even when he wasn't with me, he wanted to be. He loved my humor, my laugh and my innocence. He said he still smiles when he thinks about me. The little things we did together meant a lot to him. I asked him why it took so long to get over me. He said because in his heart, his love for me was forever and if he was honest, he doesn't know if he is completely over me after all these years. He said I was his first real love and up to this day, he has never loved someone like he loved me. He said he wished he could have been with me to take care of me when I had breast cancer. He said knowing how our relationship ended, he would have done it all over again because the time he had with me was special.

I cried after receiving his texts. Sometimes information exes give to each other can be so eye opening. It helps bring closure that some of us really need. I told him I probably took the wrong door. I never truly let our love blossom. I told him he was a sweet man and I really wish I had appreciated him and knew what I had in him. I told him his wife and family are lucky to have him. I don't think his wife would appreciate him reaching out to me, but I do hope he told her about me and that she is ok with him reaching out to me.

I continued dating Nate and it started getting serious. I ended up getting pregnant. It was so crazy when I found out that I started crying. I was devastated. I was too young to have a baby. I was having the time of my life and I wasn't ready for a baby yet. I was only 25, still young and dumb. We talked about it, and he was fine with me doing whatever I wanted to do. He already had a daughter from a previous relationship from high school. I don't think I told my family or friends about it. I didn't want anyone to change my mind or make me feel bad about my decision. I set up an appointment, we went, and I had an abortion. I think I was so frightened to bring a child into the world. I mean I still felt like a child in some aspects of my life. I was so naive. I was enjoying my life, being engaged, planning the wedding not wanting to worry about getting fat. I was just scared. I always go back in my head and wonder "what if" I had taken that other door? "What if" I would have had my baby? What would he or she look like? What would they have accomplished in this world? Would I still be Nate? Could that child have been the glue that kept us together? Woulda… Coulda… Shoulda and too many what ifs. I do have to say that getting an abortion was my biggest regret in my life. It was my one and only chance to have brought a new life into the world, given a piece of me to this crazy world. I would always tell myself that if I ever got pregnant again, no matter what the circumstance, I would have my baby. But that moment never came.

Nate and I moved in together. We had a great house in Scripps Ranch that was attached to a fault line, so that was always a little scary. Thank God, San Diego usually just got the aftershocks of earthquakes. We were engaged. My ring was beautiful. It was a marquee with two sapphire stones. I love the blue on each side of the diamond. I have never been really big on jewelry, so I didn't need a huge 5 carat ring. But it was still about a carat and a half. We didn't have a date set to get married. We were just enjoying being engaged. I told my family and friends. It was so exciting! My dad and stepmother wanted to have an engagement party for me. It was like I was big news in my small hometown. I was marrying an NFL football player. "Ricki" had made it big. That was my nickname when I was a little girl. They took an ad out in the local paper with a picture of us announcing our engagement. My relationship with my dad and stepmom was good at the time. I talked with them monthly. Nate didn't call my dad for my hand in marriage, but I didn't think I had that kind of relationship with my father. They didn't even meet my fiancé until that weekend. I think that bothered my dad since that is the traditional way but I never thought we had a traditional family. My relationship with my mother was also pretty good also. I am a forgiving person and I know she did the best she could when I was growing up. I know she didn't have any good role models in her life. Her mother was an alcoholic and abusive. She never met her father, so she didn't have a good example of love in her life from either parent. She was beautiful and smart, but she was never given the opportunity to strive when she was younger. She was a great seamstress, and a great cook, but never had the drive for more. She would get what she thought was love from the men in her life. When the drugs and alcohol took over, that was a whole other issue.

My whole family pretty much came together for my engagement party in New York. I wanted Nate to be comfortable, so we invited his mother to come with us. She is a southern lady from Moultrie, Georgia. She has six kids and Nate didn't know his dad. She raised all the kids alone, chewed snuff and talked with a thick country accent. Sometimes, it was hard to understand what she was saying.

She was very sweet to me, and I liked all five of his siblings. They all lived either in the same area or lived with their mom in the house Nate bought. We got to New York and stayed with my dad and stepmom. She had given my mom a blank check to get whatever she needed for the cookout. Everyone was getting along with one another. I always wanted my family to blend for the sake of the family. The only family member who didn't make it was my stepbrother. My stepsister came in from Los Angeles. She had met Nate since we lived only a couple of hours away and we always had a pretty good relationship.

My dad and stepmom tried to make Nate's mom as comfortable as they could living on the mountain. The water had a sulfur taste to it. We were used to it, but they made sure they had bottled water and anything else they thought would make her comfortable. We had a dinner reception at the Eagle Nest, the restaurant on top of the hill that had the best view. My friends and family had come out to celebrate my engagement. We had a great time. The next day we had the cookout at the house. My mom did most of the cooking. It was a great day mixing and mingling with more family and friends while introducing my fiancé. I was very happy. All I ever wanted was my family to come together for special occasions, enjoy one another's company and grow as a family unit.

My sister sat with Nate's mom, who began talking about my stepsister, saying she smelled like sausage. She was wearing a jean skirt. I didn't realize my future mother-in-law was racist. She didn't like white people and thought they all smelled like sausage, but she was from the deep south of Georgia. She had grown up in the civil rights era. I can't even remember if Nate had told her that my stepmom and stepsister were white. Everything would have been ok if my sister didn't go running back to my stepmom and telling what Nate's mother said. I could have killed my sister. She is such a troublemaker. She couldn't wait to say something because she knew my stepmom would go crazy. She confronted her daughter and started smelling her, which totally embarrassed her. It was just ridiculous. We all knew that our stepmom cherished her daughter and to have someone whom she invited into her house talk shit about her daughter, was pushing a button.

I said to my sister, "Why couldn't you just keep that to yourself? You just had to start some shit. We can never have a family gathering without some drama." She replied, "I thought she should know that her daughter stinks." My stepsister and one of my other friends left. She felt so embarrassed and just had to get out of there and I couldn't blame her. Shit, I wanted to get the hell out of there. I expressed to my stepmom and stepsister how sorry I was about what happened and if I had known anything like this would happen I would have never invited her. Obviously, the rest of the trip was all downhill from there. Thank God we were leaving the next day.

I went back to school full-time for interior design. I always had an eye for design and wanted to help others with their home designs. I quit working at the strip club and started shopping for my wedding gown. Things were going great and then Nate got traded from the Chargers. He had just signed a new deal with them. He was the starting wide receiver and this was going to be his best deal. He had fought for the number 2 spot so it hit him pretty hard because he thought we would be in San Diego for another 4 years. He left a piece of himself in San Diego. The rest of his career was downhill from there because that's the way the business goes. The NFL stands for "Not For Long". It's not a family; it's a business. Nobody is looking out for you but yourself and hopefully your agent. He got traded to the Los

Angeles Rams. Training camp was just two hours north. He went and got cut. His heart was broken. He wasn't focused. Finally, he got picked up by the Chicago Bears. He played special teams and he was the 3rd or 4th receiver. This was supposed to be the year he was really going to shine. He had the number 2 spot, but it was all taken instantly. He was never a starter again. That year, I stayed in California and visited on weekends while I was going to school. It was hard but we made it work. Chicago was freezing during football season, but I loved going to the games at Soldier Field. If you love football, this was a great stadium. The next year, he signed with the Atlanta Falcons so we decided to sell our home in California to move to Atlanta. He was from Moultrie, Georgia, about three hours south and all his family was there. Atlanta was a new exciting city on the rise with a great cost of living. We decided to get married there and make it our new home. We found a house and started planning the wedding. Everything was working out. I found and bought my wedding dress in San Diego. It was a beautiful sweetheart neckline with long sleeves, lace and taffeta. It was a straight dress with a train that could be added on for the ceremony and taken off for the reception. We got married at the Ritz Carlton downtown. It was a small ceremony for about 80 people. We had our mothers stand up for us. My father walked me down the aisle. My stepmother and my stepsister didn't make it to the wedding. There was still an open wound from the engagement party that was pretty depressing, but it was still a beautiful day. We ended the night leaving in a hail of bubbles. We hopped into the horse and buggy and took our carriage ride through the streets of Atlanta. The day was like a fairy tale. I had my prince charming. I got my happily ever after.

Nate went to training camp for the Atlanta Falcons that year and ended up getting cut. He would sign back with Chicago

Bears again and that would be his last season. I think he was broken when he first got traded from the Chargers. He just wasn't the same. He didn't have a Plan B and any advice I offered came off unreceived. We grew apart. I tried to get him to go to counseling but that didn't work either. Our first-year anniversary wasn't very happy and I was devastated. My happily ever after was turning into a nightmare and there was nothing I could do. You can't make someone love you or want to work on their marriage if they don't want to. He wasn't happy with himself and a little depression set in. He would tell me he wanted to take his ship down by himself and that he just didn't want to be married anymore. I was at least glad that I'd gotten a job as a flight attendant. We would have been able to survive. Yes, we would have had to downsize. He could have gotten a job as a coach, a personal trainer, and worked for Reebok... something... but No! He just wanted out and asked me for a divorced while I was in flight attendant training. He said that we would be better off as friends.

I graduated from my flight attendant training and I still had him pin my wings on me. I really thought we would be ok, but that was short lived. He didn't want to be with me. I had to just let him go. I didn't tell anyone in my family what was going on. I was embarrassed that I could barely stay married for a year. I thought that I had found my ride or die but maybe it was just our karma coming back to bite both of us in the ass. Our foundation wasn't as strong as I thought it was. When I look back, we probably shouldn't have even gotten married. He was going through the worst part of this life with his career. I already felt a bit of a pull from him during the wedding planning stages, but I thought we would be ok. I already had the dress, the wedding planner, and the venue. I couldn't cancel the wedding. That would have been devastating and embarrassing.

But there we were, a year later, and that's exactly what I was... devastated and embarrassed that I couldn't save my marriage.

I didn't contest the divorce. I didn't even tell my parents or any of my family about it until much later. They were upset that I didn't at least try to get some more furniture, my car paid for or something more than what I had taken. I just took my clothes, some household items, most of the wedding presents, a bedroom suite and the leased Z3 BMW. I had that until the lease was up. The divorce was finalized that April but I didn't move out of the house until July. I just stayed in the other bedroom. I remember driving away from the house, one last time, crying like a big ole baby and feeling like a failure. I was now a divorcee.

After my divorce, I moved in with my girlfriend Carla who had also moved to Atlanta from California. That is where we first met through my sister, when we used to go roller skating. We had so much fun. I had so many great times in San Diego. It was such a pretty city. I would love to go to the beach and just go rollerblading on the Broadway or lay out in the sun. It was such a beautiful coastline. The beach was my happy place.

It was nice to have Carla in Atlanta because I didn't have many friends since I was new to the city. I started to revert to my old ways. I reconnected with some boyfriends from my past, and started partying, drinking, and smoking again. I had quit smoking after I got married. I went to get hypnotized, and it really worked. I can still hear the crushing of the pack of cigarettes in my head. It worked because I wanted to quit. I was hoping we would have had a baby our first year, but that didn't happen. It's funny because I was waiting to have a baby after I had gotten married. I was trying to do it the right way. I looked

FREE ME 2 BE ME

back on a few years earlier when I had an abortion, wondering if that baby would have held our marriage together. I wondered if it would have been something he could have looked forward to. But woulda... coulda... shoulda... It just wasn't meant to be. I recently googled my ex-husband since he finally stopped reaching out to me after he married again. He wasn't on social media but there were a couple of stories about him. He had gained so much weight as a truck driver and he had gotten in the boxing ring for an NFL event during a Super Bowl. I was shocked to see what he looked like. I also found a YouTube video about him and his new wife talking about the concussions he received over the years and how he was experiencing the effects of the blows he had taken. The bad headaches, the depression, and the pain almost caused him to get divorced again. I don't even know if he would totally remember me if I saw him again. It was very sad. I wanted to reach out to his mother or sister just to check on him but I had lost contact with them years ago. I hope the new protocols and treatment plans the NFL has set up for their retired players is helping to take care of him. He was my 1st husband, my 1st true love. I will always have love for him.

I met another party girl named Maria. We went to all the hot parties together. This was when Atlanta was on and poppin'. She had some good hookups to get in the clubs for free. We never had to pay for anything. She didn't drink or smoke. She was just high on life and a little crazy. She didn't need anything. I drank enough for both of us on certain nights. I bought my cigarettes, cloves or Black & Milds from the lady in the bathroom. I turned into a closet smoker. We were out that night when all that stuff with Ray Lewis went down. It's funny I met Ray in San Diego when the Super Bowl was there. He was just getting into the league and wasn't the big star he had become by the time everything happened. A couple of girlfriends, his friend and I spent the day in Tijuana. We had a great time drinking corona and tequila shots. That was during a time when you could walk across the border. We used to go to Tijuana to party for cheap. It was so wild and crazy. The tequila shots were the best. The servers went around with a bottle and a whistle, tilt your head back, poured tequila in your mouth, shut it, put their hand over your mouth, blew the whistle while shaking your head at the same time, and then threw your head forward. We got so fucked up.

Maria and I were out in Buckhead when Wolf, Puffy's bodyguard, was shot and killed. This was when BMF was running the city. Thank God, I wasn't into drug dealers. They always scared me. I always thought of them as abusers and that they had to have control over you. I wasn't a controllable woman so I couldn't be persuaded by just money or drugs. Atlanta is so different now. The clubs close a couple hours earlier at 2 a.m. and Buckhead is now the Rodeo Drive of the south... or at least it's trying to be. I haven't been out to party like I used to party in years now. It's just for birthday celebrations or brunch. My friendship with Maria turned into her becoming my best friend. We used to talk every day. I haven't spoken to her in over three years now. It's so crazy how your life evolves and the different direction it starts to take when you get older. I missed her a lot in the beginning, but not so much now. When you can step out of a relationship (be it with a girlfriend or a boyfriend) you can see things so clearly. I believe any relationship needs to have open communication; it can't be a one-way street. If I can't say something... anything... to my best friend, offer advice or share my opinion, or disagree on any topic, then what kind of friendship is that? You can't just be giving people advice and then not be able to take advice or criticism about your own life, thinking that you can always solve your own problems. It's got to be open communication on both sides. If you don't like something I said, tell me, curse me out or say thank you, but I know what I am doing. So, instead of having a conversation with me, she uses social media to make a comment about our conversation saying be careful about what you tell others; they will use it against you.

When I saw it, I was like, "Really?" I tried calling her phone with no answer and I haven't talked to her since then. I know something else was going on with her. We had our first problem within our relationship right before my 40th birthday. She didn't show up to any of my birthday gatherings. She had asked me to lend her some money to pay her rent. She knew that I had just gotten some money from my boyfriend and asked to borrow it. Over the course of our friendship, I had previously taken out a loan for her so she could take care of some debt. She would pay me back on a monthly basis until the loan was paid off, but I would almost always have to ask her for the payment. On other occasions, I would buy her a purse or other items at Macy's and put them on my card. She would pay me back so it never really bothered me. But one time she told me that I didn't have kids or anyone else to take care of and that I probably didn't even need the money. What? I don't need my own money? That statement hurt because now I felt like she was taking advantage of/using me. After she paid me back the last time, I said to myself that I am never loaning money to her again. When she asked for money to pay her rent, I felt bad. I am a very giving person and I know times can get tough taking care of two boys pretty much by herself. But I felt like she had boyfriends who should have been helping her, not me.

When I got divorced, I didn't receive a lump sum of money from

ERIKA WEATHERS

Nate. He was practically broke except for his 401k savings. I started using my credit cards to pay my bills and ended up getting myself in debt. I finally got myself together and worked on paying off my debt. I improved my credit score and vowed never to have debt problems again. I still maintain that goal. I worked hard to get my score into the high 800s. So, I told Maria I was her friend not a bank. I told her that if I loaned her the money, it would be the last time. She didn't like that. She didn't take the money and stopped talking to me. About a year went by and she reached out to me and apologized. She had a lot going on with her boys and just wasn't in a good place so pushing away was what she needed at the time. She was now pregnant with her third child and had probably gotten pregnant around my 40th birthday. I was at the hospital when she had her baby girl. We were back to being friends, but it wasn't the same. She was there to celebrate my 45th birthday but that next year, right before her birthday, we had a conversation about her grown boys – one was away after graduating college and the other was getting ready to get out of jail. I was just giving her my advice on how to deal with both situations. I told her that sometimes tough love had to be applied. She had many positive times with them but was simply experiencing some negatives.

Because I don't have children, some people will say, "What do you know?", But I was a kid before. You can't continue to spoil your kids and not let them see the consequences of their actions. You can't continue to save them. You must let them live. But that's just me and how I would have parented if I had kids. My response to her on social media was a quote from Dr. Suess: ``Be who you are and say what you feel because those who mind don't matter and those who matter don't mind."

FREE ME 2 BE ME

Money is the root of most evils but words can cut you to the core. I never meant any ill will nor was I trying to put anyone down. I was just voicing my opinions on what I had seen over the course of our 10+ years of friendship. It had grown in so many ways. We were girls that were becoming women, but I believed that I had outgrown the friendship. I couldn't stand being on the phone sometimes listening to the same stories over and over again, never able to get in a word, just agreeing to let it play out. I knew when we had started to talk again it was never going to be the same because I wasn't the same. I had grown. I wanted more from the friendship and she was still worried about posting half-naked pictures or getting liposuction or fat injections trying to keep up with the younger girls being at the "in" parties. I had just outgrown it. She was stuck, plus had a young girl to raise. I needed more. I had to realize, in all my relationships, I had to put myself first. I had survived two bouts with breast cancer. Shit, I survived just living in general. I am a survivor. My survivorship is what matters. I had to come first.

1. How is your relationship with your parents? With your siblings?

_____
_____
_____

2. Do you still have friends from your childhood?

_____
_____
_____

3. Who is your best friend and what do you love most about them?

_____
_____
_____

4. Do you have a good credit score? Is that important to you? Why or Why not?

_____
_____
_____

5. Who gave you a helping hand and how has that impacted your life?

_____
_____
_____

> *"There is no gain without some pain. I will continue to work hard to get my result. I may be getting older, but I'm also getting bolder. I know I can do it….never doubt me. Here I come!"*

CHAPTER THREE

WHAT THE HELL

Cancer: a malignant tumor of potentially unlimited growth that expands locally by invasion and systemically by metastasis.

ERIKA WEATHERS

I was 33 years old when I found out I had breast cancer. I really couldn't believe it. Sometimes, I would ask myself, "Why me? What did I do?" I had seen ads and commercials about breast cancer but thought you couldn't get it until you were in your 60s. I never thought it would be me. I didn't know anybody who had breast cancer but now that I had it, I had met so many people with cancer that are all younger than 60. But just like everything in life, you don't pay attention until something affects you... touches you. I never thought about the consequences and how the way you live your life can come back and rock your world. We think we are invincible. We live our lives trying to figure out what we are going to do with ourselves. Then that five-year plan you set for yourself gets interrupted and you have to press pause. You have to map out a new path until you can jump back on your road to your success. They say 1-in-8 women have breast cancer and it can happen as early as their 20s, not the typical 60s I thought. The times have changed. Our world is not the same with new technologies, pesticides, pollution, hormones and antibiotics all affecting the diseases, viruses and cancers we come in contact with.

I have always had lumpy breasts and very dense with lots of cysts but never had any worries until I felt a lump in my right breast that felt a little different from the norm. In 2001, I went in for my annual appointment. My doctor felt a couple of lumps in my breast that he wanted further tests on. He sent me for a needle biopsy. They found three different size masses: one small, one medium, and one large. They put them all in the same family and did a biopsy on the largest mass. The doctor said that I have dense breast which means fibrous and glandular. There's not much fatty tissue present and millions of cysts making things look more suspicious. They just wanted to check to make sure everything was ok. The results came back benign which was great news at the time.

The next year, I had to find a new doctor because my old one had moved out of state. I went in for my annual checkup. She looked over my test results from my previous exams and wanted me to get an ultrasound on my breast to make sure nothing had changed. During the exam, they measured the previous masses and found that the smallest of the three had grown and they wanted me to do another needle biopsy on that mass. I was a little hesitant at first but my mom told me to make an appointment right away. The results came back and the doctor called me to the office. I knew that wasn't a good sign. Just tell me. It doesn't matter if I'm in front of you or at home. Just make sure I'm not driving which was the protocol, at least the first time.

I took my best friend (at the time) with me and we waited for the doctor to come in. He told me I had cancer. I mean I knew what he was going to say but to hear the big "C" made me start crying. My best friend started crying, too. I gathered myself and tried to listen to what he was saying.

Dang! I was only 33 years old, in the prime of my life, in the best shape of my life or so I thought. I was single and having the time of my life in Atlanta and then to learn I have cancer. It was all happening in slow motion... Thoughts were on repeat in my mind. Why me? What did I do to deserve this? Was I going to lose my breast? My hair? Was I going to look sick? Why? OMG? Will I die?

I went to see a surgeon and plastic surgeon to find out what I needed to do to get the cancer out of me. The first doctor had me get a mammogram and told me that I had lobular cancer. He gave me options of getting a full mastectomy and a lift or having both breasts removed just in case the cancer spread to the other breast because of the type of cancer it was. My first thought was to just have both breasts removed and get implants and reconstructive surgery with my areola and nipples tattooed on. I went to the plastic surgeon, he measured my breasts, showed me the implants and told me about the procedure. I didn't like the plastic surgeon at all. He treated me like a number, not a person. It was almost like he wasn't even listening to what I wanted. On top of that, the doctors suggested the double mastectomy. He wanted to set a date because they were moving offices and it needed to be done before then. Really? So, I needed to work around both of their schedules and remove both breasts just in case it came back in the other breast... without a second opinion. They didn't want to give me time to think about what if the cancer never spread to my other breast. I was like no sir! I was so pissed with both doctors. Neither had a good bedside manner. I knew I needed to get a second opinion because I knew I couldn't work with these two!

I fired those guys and sought a second opinion from another doctor who could remove the cancer *and* be my plastic surgeon to reconstruct my new breasts. His name was Dr. Grant Carlson. What a great name for a doctor, right? I'm glad I did. He told me the cancer I had was not the cancer I was told I had. I had ductal carcinoma situ, more specifically infiltrating ductal carcinoma grade 1 ca slow growing stage 1 with negative nodes 1.2cm ER & PR positive Her2+. We decided on a full mastectomy because the cancer was close to my inner wall and a lumpectomy would leave me deformed and may not remove all the cancer.

My surgery was scheduled for August 14, 2003, five days before my 34th birthday. So, my right breast was removed and I had a lift on my left so it would be at the same level as the right one once it fell. They also checked to see if the cancer spread to any other part of my body. They removed 13 lymph nodes. All were tested and all came back negative. That was great news. Thank the Lord!

The day after my surgery, I was sent home with a drain hanging out of me where 13 lymph nodes were removed. All of my breast tissue and my nipple were taken, and a tissue expander placed in my chest cavity. Thank God my mom was there to help me take care of the daily removal of the drainage. YUCK!

It had been several weeks since my surgery. I was still a little numb under my arm. I had gotten the last of my injections into my tissue expander. It was so hard. I had been trying to push the expander to the left to fill in the empty space because it was sitting more under my armpit, so I had to massage it into my chest cavity. I also had to start massaging my scar tissue from where they cut my lymph nodes, so the lumps didn't stay or keloid. I had to leave the expander in for three months so my skin and chest muscle could stretch. I remember having my hair braided to the back so I didn't have to worry about doing it. That's my ride or die look. My birthday present that year was that my lymph nodes were clear. No more cancer because they had gotten it all. Thank the Lord! Praise God!! I knew that I was truly blessed having found the cancer before it had grown or spread. Through the whole process I tried to stay strong and confident thinking that everything would be alright. I think the only time I really cried was when I got my second opinion from Dr. Carlson. It felt like I was really getting ready to go through a major life-changing event. I had been telling everybody that I had cancer, even joking a little about it. I guess I did it to make it easier for others. The next step was to wait for all my tests to come back so I could find out my treatment plan. All my lymph nodes were negative, my hormone receptors came back positive, and my fish test (DNA) came back negative, which were all good. I thought I wouldn't need chemo but when I met with the oncologist, he recommended that I start taking the tamoxifen for five years and three months of chemo, four cycles every three weeks. I was very disappointed I had gotten this far and my mind was getting a little crazy. I really didn't want to put poison into my body knowing it would kill my good and bad cells. I would lose my hair, be fatigued and look sick. It would have been the worst part of the whole ordeal. My oncologists conferred with each other and felt that I didn't need chemotherapy or radiation because I was ER+ and PR+. They felt that neither would have helped me and instead suggested putting me on the tamoxifen, which is an estrogen blocker with a bunch of side-effects like blood clots, stroke, endometrial cancer, hot flashes, loss of libido, vaginal dryness, depression, mood swings... Should I go on? There are so many more.

In my mid-30s with no libido, a dry pussy and only one good boob... my sex life was over! Only a small percent of women get the side effects and most just get a few of them. It wasn't like I had a man in my life at the time anyway. I knew that I was blessed to be alive and that I would figure it out. Plus, I didn't need chemotherapy! Hallelujah! It was such a big relief but my oncologist wanted me to get the size of my uterus checked to make sure it wasn't swollen. She wanted a genetic test to make sure I didn't have the gene, or she was going to gut me and take my ovaries and uterus. I didn't look sick and if you didn't know me, you wouldn't have known what I just went through.

I found out that day I was allergic to morphine. I would start to cry, then start to laugh, almost pissing on myself. My mom was like what is wrong with you? It was so crazy; it was like I was crazy. They took me off of that pain medicine and sent me home with Percocet. I had pain but it wasn't unbearable. I have a pretty good pain threshold. I would only take one pill but it didn't do anything for me so I started taking two pills at a time as prescribed and they made me feel so good. I liked them. They helped me relax and sleep. I see how people can get addicted if you're not careful. You really have to wean yourself off of them. For my birthday that year, I had some friends come over. Pat bought a big tub of ice cream and cake. It was so good. You can never go wrong with cake and ice cream. It brought back some normalcy to my life that was much appreciated.

After healing for a couple months, we started the reconstruction process. The tissue expander placed in my breast during my surgery would be replaced with my implant in about six months. I would go in monthly and have saline injected into my breast to stretch it. There really wasn't much pain but over the course of injections my breast would grow a little at a time. It was funny. I remember having a Barbie doll when I was younger whose breasts would grow when you turned her arm so you could make them go from being flat chested to being a full C! I had to see the humor in everything. It made it so much easier. I was a real life Barbie doll getting my breast reconstructed. I chose to get the silicone gel implants even though they were not being sold to the public at the time. If you needed reconstructive surgery, you could choose between the silicone gel implants or the saline. I wanted it to look and feel more like my natural breast. They closely mimicked the feel of human fat. My other options were to use my own fat to build a boob out of my own tissues. I didn't really have enough fat. Some women use their belly flat and it's almost like getting a tummy tuck. I really didn't want any extra cuts or scars on my belly or back anyway. They call that the trap flap. I was also too young to not have reconstruction. I am too vain to have a concave flat chest. I knew that wasn't an option for me but God bless the women who have made that choice. I had my implant put in and at the same time, my left breast was lifted and my areola was cut smaller. I wanted to keep one real natural boob no implant, no removal of that breast. I just wanted my boob! I refer to them as my good boob and my implant.

One of my friends said, "Oh, at least you can get a boob job now." I was like, "Really?" I know my face looked like, "Are you stupid, Bitch? Don't you think if I wasn't happy with my boobs that I would have gotten a boob job a long time ago?" No one wants to be a part of the cancer club, but when you become a part of it, you do what you have to do to survive. Really ladies, please think before you speak. I had cancer. I had to have my breast removed. I had to get an implant to look normal again. Really, please stop. Don't say that to another survivor because it hasn't just been one lady that said this to me. But still, I just smile because I know you don't really know what to say. Next time, just don't say anything or how about "I'm sorry you had to go through that at such a young age and you are blessed to still be here." That sounds pretty good, right? Ok vent over.

The next step in the reconstruction process was getting my areola tattooed and adding my new nipple. They cut me right above my bikini line almost like a C-section. Only a smaller cut removed some skin and formed that skin into a nipple and attached it to the center of my areola. So my nipple would always be hard. I would wear a wireless padded bra so my one nipple wouldn't show through. Over time, the nipple would flatten out because it was just tissue with nothing inserted to keep it erect. Nowadays, they have new techniques: nipple sparing, 3D tattooing, and better nipple construction so that it stays erect and looks more natural. With all the money for research to find a cure, at least they are finding ways for women to hold on to their breasts without having to lose them completely. The research money seems to go toward finding better forms of chemo, localization of radiation, and hormonal therapies. They still can't find a cure after all these years, but at least women have more choices and better options to look as normal and natural as possible. I was pretty happy with my results. The tattoo and nipple covered most of my scar. I was still almost a C when I had my bra on. My breast looked pretty good. I started putting lightening cream on my scar to try to make it blend and fade. Since I didn't need chemo or radiation, I started taking the hormonal therapy Tamoxifen. The protocol was to take it for five years. I took it for two years because the side effects made me bitchier than I normally was, and it caused me to gain weight. I had to work out just to maintain that weight. I always felt bloated and my clothes fit tighter. It didn't stop my period; it just turned it into a 40-day cycle with no early menopause. I had bouts of depression and feelings of being less of a woman. I had thoughts that now no one would want me when they could have a woman with both of their breasts. I just had a lot of self-doubt. Tamoxifen is an estrogen blocker so it was supposed to stop my period but it didn't, which was another reason my cancer mutated at such a young age. The estrogen had always been pumping in my body. After I stopped taking it, it eventually left my system and I started feeling like my old self again... like I never had cancer.

I got a new oncologist who wanted me to get the gene test to make sure I didn't have the BRCA gene. If I did, she recommended to remove my ovaries, my other breast, my uterus and Fallopian tubes... everything! I would also go into menopause. My God! I began feeling like less than a woman again. I played all of these mind games with myself.

The test came back negative. I didn't have the gene. WHEW! Thank you again God! I didn't have any kids yet and that was still a possibility for me. I stopped seeing my oncologist because she was getting ready to move to Chicago. She was my favorite. My last oncologist had no personality or bedside manner so since I was off my medication, I would just see Dr. Carlson annually and rotate my mammogram and breast MRI every six month.

1. What is the worst news you received in your life? How did you handle it?

_____
_____
_____

2. Are you open to asking for help when needed? Why or Why not?

_____
_____
_____

3. What is the best news you received in your life? How did you handle it?

_____
_____
_____

FREE ME 2 BE ME

4. Do you go to the doctor for regular checkups? If no, why not?

_____
_____
_____

5. What bad habits do you have? Do you want to change them? If no, why not?

_____
_____
_____

> *"Time waits for no one. Life is too short. Make the most of it now and stop waiting for everything to be just right. Live your moments now."*

CHAPTER FOUR

LOVE THYSELF

Value: To be worthy or rate highly, cherish, consider precious, the importance or usefulness of something. Standards of behavior.

ERIKA WEATHERS

We don't get to pick our family, so you do the best you can and hope you turn out ok. I think I turned out ok. Shit, I know I turned out better than ok. I knocked on the door to my 50s, and I walked right in. I still can't believe it. I'm single, divorced, no kids, some good girlfriends, ok relationship with family and a two-time breast cancer survivor. I celebrated being 13 years cancer free on June 3, 2021! I have been a flight attendant for over 20 years. I thought I would be able to retire in five years, with lifetime free flight benefits on Delta, but all that went out the window since finding out that our contract has been cancelled. My future with my company is unknown. I'm just riding it out, praying and hoping we get bought by one of the majors or at least get another contract and our union gets it together to merge our seniority list.

Well, United bought our company, but only 49% of it. So there is no more flying for Delta and American. We were waiting on the company and our union to come together on a new contract that the flight attendants would approve or have an arbitrator come in and stamp a fair deal for both sides. Well, the arbitrator finally came to the table and stamped the last contract that was offered to us. My seniority will be restored. It took less than a year. I was only on reserve for six months. I got a little raise but at the end of the day, I am happy where I am. I am glad that I stuck it out and stayed. Granted, the regional airlines don't pay as much money as the major airlines, but I struggled with leaving over the years, especially with everything we just went through with contract negotiations and losing Delta and American contracts. It was scary that we could have lost everything. A lot of my friends did leave for other airlines, but when you switch airlines, you lose your seniority and usually take a pay cut. They had to start over and wait about five years to get back to making a decent living. That is a lot of pressure so

FREE ME 2 BE ME

late in life.

I am now in my 50s, still single and not even in the mood to date. I'm trying to figure out this second half of my life. My new normal was commuting to work, which meant flying from Atlanta to start my trip out of my new base Chicago, Illinois. Commuter life hasn't been too bad. I can take a nap going and coming if I need to. It's changed my life but not dramatically. I got a Crash Pad with about 13 other flight attendants all working for different airlines. I did have a couple of friends from my airlines there. We all paid $135 a month, which is very reasonable. Other flight attendants were paying $250 to $350 a month, so we really had a steal. A crash pad is a hotel room with bunk beds and a couple of full size beds. We are not all there at the same time. We make a calendar for the month so that we can see if we will need to get another room. We only allow 4 girls in the room a night and it usually works out well because some flight attendants are on reserve and others have lines. With that, some ladies are only there once or twice a month and some are there 10 days a month. But even with just staying for one night, the $135 is worth it, especially for the peace of mind to be able to come in a day before your trip or to stay the night after your trip.

After being on reserve, not knowing my schedule, and being on call for 5 to 6 days, I couldn't wait to get my seniority back. With seniority, I could bid commutable trips, get back on a good workout schedule, back in my acting classes and maybe find a man to share my life with. Oh to dream! I got back my seniority, a pay raise and better trips and then COVID hit. In a matter of 6 months, my company was shutting down operations and we lost our contract with United. It was crazy! We had made it through all the contract negotiations and finally started seeing the light at the end of the tunnel just to be slapped in the face hard. I would tell my friends that it was like a bad relationship with a boyfriend. We had our ups and downs but I decided to stay and ride it out hoping it would get better. Then, his ass breaks up with me. I probably should have been gone from my job years ago and working with a major airline. I should have broken up with my boyfriend a year and half into it, instead of staying for another year waiting for him to break up with me. I just get comfortable in situations and hope for the best. Well, that doesn't work. I need to take control of my life.

The fifth chapter has begun; it's 2021. I became an official poll worker, working the U.S. Senate runoff elections in Georgia and hoping for a win with Jon Ossoff and Rev. Raphael Warnock so President Joe Biden can get our country turned around. With him, would come better healthcare, getting the pandemic under control, an improved economy, police reform... and the list goes on. I am also now a notary. I got my embossed stamp. I will finish my associate's degree in criminal justice by the end of the year. I attended real estate school in March and got my license in May. Now I need to find a broker to work with. I just joined NPU-Unit M, my Neighborhood Planning Unit. I am the secretary getting more involved in my community working with the police, city council and community members so we can voice our concerns on matters in our neighborhood.

I'm also an aspiring actress. I have booked a cable TV reenactment show, indie projects, local commercials and some industrials. I'm hoping to book a union gig on TV or film or a SAG commercial soon. I really need to continue to work on my craft by training on a regular basis. I also have to increase my confidence that I can do it! After losing my job as a flight attendant, I thought I had retired my wings. But I missed it, so I applied with an airline here in Atlanta. It was actually the same company that took over for us when Delta canceled our contract, so I got my wings back. I was back in my same break room. It was so surreal. Maybe I'll get these flying benefits with Delta after all! With endless possibilities for my future, I can't wait to see all the doors continuing to open for me.

I have always wanted to write a book to help those young girls in grade school, high school, college or just that girl who needs a direction or a mentor to push her and give her motivation. I so needed that when I was coming up. With all of the technology and different avenues available to kids nowadays they already have an upper hand but some still don't know how to take advantage of it or really know what they need. If I could help just one girl that would mean the world to me because just one could turn into hundreds.

I lived with my mom growing up, who was single and working as a bartender. She wasn't home most nights, so my place would turn into a hangout for my friends. We had some great parties. We always found a way to get alcohol and drugs. It amazes me what we got away with at such a young age. I remember my sweet sixteen party. We had a keg. Yes, so crazy! That night was like a scene from the movie Sixteen Candles. A couple friends and I were getting high in a red Trans Am, opening the door and a bunch of smoke following behind us. We were so high. And, yes this party was supervised by our parents. All of my girlfriends had gotten the same dress but different animal prints on it. At the end of the night, we were wearing T-shirts and shorts. One of my girlfriends was date raped that night. She didn't tell any of us until several years later. We felt that she was acting differently, but we would have never expected that such a horrible act would have happened to her, especially when she was still a virgin. I am so glad that she told us, dealt with the ordeal and didn't let the violent act rule her life.

I didn't get a lot of direction from my mom. She didn't take great interest in my schooling or come watch me participate in any of my extracurricular activities. In high school, I wished I had a better coach, guidance counselor or teacher to take an interest in me and see I was a good athlete. I used to beat most of the boys in grade school and I was the fastest sprinter in high school. I only started running track because there was a cute Black guy with green eyes who ran. I almost made it to states that year missing it by seconds... literally seconds. I was that good. Imagine, if I had taken it seriously and trained properly (no smoking cigarettes, smoking weed and drinking) during the season, I could have possibly gotten a scholarship. I didn't see the possibilities. No adult in my life took interest in me, not even my track coach. Was it because I was Black? Was it because he just didn't give a shit? Was he just there for a paycheck? He wasn't even in shape himself, so how could I expect him to take it seriously? I needed someone to step up in my life to be my mentor, but they never came. I didn't know any better. I didn't even really think about going to college. Who would pay for it? Who could I become if I went? There were so many questions but no real answers. I didn't have a real focus for the future. It just was never on my radar. I didn't worry about the SAT's, looking at colleges, or even thinking about my future. I just wanted out of New York and I would figure everything else out later.

I remember going to my guidance counselor but not getting any guidance. My grades were above average but back then, there was racism. Excuse me a second. There is still racism, it just rears its head in different ways today. Back then, they didn't

FREE ME 2 BE ME

want to help the Black kids. There weren't too many of us but they didn't have high hopes for us. It was like we should just be happy to be graduating with a high school diploma. I remember one time when I was going out for football cheerleading, I had already been on the team the year before. For some reason, the new coach didn't like me. It was probably because I was Black. She intimidated me so much that I messed up and didn't make the team that year.

I was put on the squad for soccer cheerleading. I felt like crap. I was so disappointed in myself for letting her get to me that I made sure I was back on the varsity squad that next year cheering for the football team. I have always loved football even when I was a little girl. I especially loved it when the Dallas Cowboys had Tony Dorsett; the Pittsburgh Steelers had Lynn Swan and Terry Bradshaw; and the Giants with Lawrence Taylor. I have always been a fan but now I'm a Cowboys hater. I just wanted to graduate and get the hell out of New York. I knew I didn't want to live in a state where it snows, so when my sister invited me to move to California to help with her kids, and to try to figure out what to do with my life, it was exactly what I did. I didn't really know my sister very well. She was six years older than me. She lived with my father but I was just happy to have a place to go. She lived in San Diego, California, with sunshine and beaches, so as soon as I saved enough money for a plane ticket and graduated from high school, I would be on that plane... gone!

In school, I was too busy smoking in the fields with friends. We used to sit and smoke a whole pack of cigarettes acting like we were doing something... getting a head rush. I was more interested in partying with friends, doing drugs and drinking. I did enough school work to pass and graduate with my high school diploma. My freshman year, I was the only child at home. My brother was four years older than me and had gone away to the Air Force. My older sister, who was six years older than me, lived with my father and went to the Navy. My twin lived with my father and went to a different high school. After graduating, he went to community college for a year and then joined the Marines. I knew I wasn't going into the Armed Forces. It just wasn't for me. I was the prissy one in the family. Living with my mother, we seemed to move every year. We moved from the townhouse, to the brown house, to the duplex, to me living with my friend and her family in my senior year because my mother couldn't afford a two bedroom. I didn't want to live with my dad my senior year because I would have had to go to a different school district. I wanted to be able to graduate with my friends and enjoy my last year in school. I would have been isolated with no extracurricular activity. The only good thing about it would have been being able to live with my twin and my stepsister. We were all the same age. We were the babies out of the six kids.

I have always used my sexuality since I was a young girl. I knew I was cute and I thought having a pretty face was all I had to offer. I went to school with mostly white kids and that's all I hung out with besides my cousin and a few other Black kids. I was mixed but I was still a Black girl. And even though I thought I fit in, I never really saw the racism all around me. I experienced parents not wanting their boys to date a Black girl, as well as some of my "friends" using the "N" word around me but saying they weren't talking about me. I was so naïve. I mean hell, I wanted to be white. I wished my name was Jennifer or Lisa and that my hair was straight and not puffy and nappy!

I did anything to fit in when I was younger. Instead of wearing

FREE ME 2 BE ME

braids, I would try to comb it out and wear it straight. I was a young Diana Ross with the big hair. I felt like I had to try and fit in most of my life. I was either too light or too dark. I always knew I was good looking but I never realized that I had a natural beauty. When I put makeup on and got my hair done, I was gorgeous. I never valued myself. I never realized that I was the prize. My self-esteem was garbage. I let others take advantage of me without being aware of the treasures I actually possessed. That was my MO (modus operandi) for years until I finally learned to love myself. But I'm still a work in progress. I still have my insecurities, self-doubt and question my self-worth. Trying to stay positive and take care of yourself is a never ending process. You just have to keep talking to yourself and say, "I am enough!" You must learn to believe in yourself because if you don't, nobody else will.

I didn't have any values. My stepmother used to tell me that my values weren't the same as hers, but she never taught me anything about values. She, my mother, and my father, simply hoped I didn't get pregnant. What I needed to hear was, "You are a precious gem. Don't let anyone take advantage of you. Love yourself. Respect yourself. Save those cookies for someone who loves you and respects you... because YOU are the prize." But I never heard any of that! It is a true blessing that I didn't end up pregnant or addicted to drugs. My life would have been totally different and I probably wouldn't have made it out of Middletown, New York. Thank God! God had a plan for me.

Because I didn't hear those things, I gave my cookies away looking for some attention, even if it was short lived until the next boy came along. All of my ill-advised escapades were done in the dark. Most of my friends didn't know who I was sleeping with... or so I thought. Most of my girlfriends were virgins or had boyfriends. We were the popular group at our high school. I was a football and soccer cheerleader and a mat maid, that's a cheerleader for wrestling. I ran track, did the long jump, and played softball. I really was a good kid. My grades were Bs and Cs. But my dark side was me being promiscuous and thinking that sleeping with different boys would make me feel better, but it didn't. I was sleeping with other girls' boyfriends, wanting what I couldn't have, and thinking that they would choose me. I didn't realize they were just taking advantage of me because they could. I really wish I knew why I did some of the things I did. Sometimes I wondered if I was ever molested when I was younger and completely blocked it out of my childhood memories. My childhood memories are not very good. I have to see pictures or hear someone tell a story to remind me. I always remember the yellow house at the bottom of the mountain. My stepmother was on top of the mountain. My dad met her when he was doing some handy work for her around the house. When we lived in the yellow house, all four kids were together. I remember pictures of me and my twin brother, at our birthday party, in our cute matching outfits. My mother also had us modeling for JCPenney. We were so adorable, if I do say so myself. We had a nice house, lots of yard space, and had food on the table. We may have been struggling but for the most part, we had a decent childhood... until our parents divorced.

I think I learned about sex in health education. I don't remember anyone telling me about the birds and the bees. We would watch movies like Sixteen Candles, Pretty in Pink, The Breakfast Club, and The Brat Pack, just to name a few of my favorites. When I was a freshman in high school, I lost my virginity to the boy I ran track with. He was a senior at the time. It wasn't a relationship; it was just a fling. I gave up my virginity to a boy I barely knew who didn't give two shits about me. He was just taking advantage of a young freshman who knew no better than to lay down and spread her legs. I was looking for love in all the wrong places. Actually, it wasn't even love I was looking for; it was attention because I didn't know what love was. That was my MO throughout high school. I didn't have a male figure in my life who gave me the love and support that I needed. So, I hooked up with different guys. I liked them but would never get what I needed or even the girlfriend title. They just used me. I was never looked at as the girlfriend and that was probably because I was Black. I never gave the guys who really liked me an opportunity. They were probably the guys who would have respected me and showed me the love I wanted.

There was a guy friend who went to school with my sister and brother in another district. He would take me out to buy me things. He was so nice and respectful to me. He never tried to take advantage of me and I wouldn't even kiss him. Everyone thought he was my boyfriend but he wasn't. I don't know why I wouldn't accept him as my boyfriend even though that's what he wanted. I remember kissing him on New Year's Eve and pulling back like it was a mistake. He should have been my high school sweetheart and first love. But I didn't give it a chance. I really don't know what was wrong with me. It was like I wanted to be treated like shit. Why would I choose that over a good, respectful relationship with someone who really cared about me? Why? How could I be that screwed up at such a young age?

That guy ended up marrying a hometown girl named Erika... yes with a K. I just wanted to be used. I was really just fucked up and damaged. I never liked the good guy, the nice guy. I always wanted the bad boy. That's what most everyone wanted: the jock, the pretty boy, or the guy who could have anyone he wanted. It's so funny, but not really.

I was voted class flirt my senior year. It could be taken that I was the class hoe and that's not really cool. I didn't take it that way. I didn't really think people thought I was a slut. I was one of the popular girls. Nobody knew what I was really doing.

I would see my father on occasions but our relationship was strained. I felt like I could never do right by him. I never felt like I was daddy's girl. He never came to any of my track meets or my softball games. He had to work to pay the bills. He wanted us to get good grades and didn't think that extracurricular activities mattered. I don't even remember my father or my mother coming to my graduation and that's just horrible. My mother said she came, but it took her forever to find parking and then she couldn't find a seat, so she just left. At least she tried, but it was expected. I probably didn't even tell my dad when it was.

I lived with my girlfriend and her family my senior year in high school. My mother couldn't afford our apartment and had to move into a one bedroom. She said I could sleep on the couch. I always thought that she did that on purpose because that was what her mother did to her. But she said it was because she didn't have any money. My friend knew what I was going through and asked her parents if I could live with them for my senior year. I really didn't want to live with my father, my stepmother, or my twin or stepsister at the time because I would have had to transfer schools and not graduate with all my friends. I would have been sheltered for my last year, so thank God my friend's parents said it was ok. I really appreciated them. I was so happy that they welcomed me into their home because they really didn't have to and they already had a house full. I shared my friend's room, her bed and her stuff. I had a part-time job and tried to not be a burden and help out where I could. My girlfriend and her family were so welcoming. I knew there had to be some good in me for the whole family to be accepting of me.

Kathy was almost totally opposite of me. She was a virgin at the time. She has only ever slept with one man, her husband. Yes, she had other boyfriends, but she waited until marriage to have sex. She is still married with three great boys that are turning into men. She has a great life. Sometimes I wonder why she looked out for me and why she made a plea to her whole family for me. I'm sitting here right now with tears in my eyes because of that great gesture she made for me. I could have taken so many bad turns in my life. So, I called her and she told me that she would do the same thing today if someone didn't have a place to live. Her parents said Kathy didn't ask; she pretty much told them I needed a place to stay and that I would be sharing her room. I was like, "Really? You just told them and they were like ok?" The whole family was a godsend. I appreciate and love them all so much. I still send and receive Christmas cards from them and visit them whenever I get a chance to go home. They still live in the same home.

I think we all probably reevaluate our lives when we hit those special milestones in life. Looking back at that little girl, Ricki, my accomplishments and failures that were met over the years have helped mold me for the new achievements and defeats of my life. And through it all, I have survived. I will continue to thrive. I have so many more milestones to hit. I have made it to this point in life as a full grown woman leaping into her 50s. We all still have that little girl or boy in us trying to escape the bad habits, behavior and awkwardness that we hoped we would have outgrown by now. We are just trying to be our authentic selves, making our way in the world and trying to find out what truly makes us happy. Looking back, you can see the potential that you had, the missed opportunities, and the crazy encounters you had along the way. We try to grow up so fast thinking that we know everything and then realize how stupid or naive we were. I have had a well-rounded life. I have done so many things. I am grateful for all the people who I have encountered along the way, even though I have been single for the majority of my life. The special relationships have gotten me ready for the one person I will spend my golden years with. If that's not in the cards and if my cousin Dawn is still single, I'll make her my travel companion and we will continue to travel the world together, laughing and farting the whole way.

1. Who was your best friend in grade school? Are you still friends today?

_____
_____
_____

2. What one thing did you like about yourself when you were young? Do you still like that thing about yourself today?

_____
_____
_____

3. What one thing did you dislike about yourself when you were young? Do you still dislike that thing about yourself today?

_____
_____
_____

4. Did you know what you wanted to be when you grew up? If yes, what was it?

_____
_____
_____

5. If you could change anything about your childhood, what would it be? Why?

_____
_____
_____

"I totally believe everything happens for a reason. Don't fight; it just let it be. Don't stress yourself over things that are out of your control. People will come in and out of your life. Just look around and see who is still there. That's all that really matters."

ERIKA WEATHERS

CHAPTER FIVE

BACK TO LIFE

Identity: The distinguishing character or personality of an individual, specification, self.

After surgery, I started eating extra healthy. I was cutting out all animal products, sugar, and caffeine. I started drinking 8 ounces of this root juice, daily, for 10 days. It looked, smelled and tasted like shit. I had to plug my nose to drink it and would almost always gag before I could get it down. It was disgusting! But it actually made me feel really good, energized and alert. It cleaned me out... if you know what I mean. It was supposed to be a cure all and clean all the bad toxins out of my body. I had also quit smoking the day before my surgery. I was really just a closet smoker, bumming cigarettes, buying Black & Milds or cloves from the bathroom attendant. I also stopped drinking. I was going to the herb shop on the regular trying all the products I researched and found in all the breast cancer books that would help me stay cancer free. The doctors can never tell you how you got the cancer but just give suggestions on what can help. Some of that stuff is expensive but you will do whatever you need to to survive. I was taking so many supplements. I was feeling good but I also started having anxiety. My heart rate would accelerate. It was from a mixture of all the supplements and all the reading I was doing on the survival of cancer: life after cancer, what to expect after surgery, and trying to understand the cause and effect of my breast cancer. It was a lot and I just had to stop reading because I was driving myself crazy.

I couldn't really start working out for almost 8 months after my surgery. I could walk and do some light activities but I had to rebuild my chest. It was a slow process. I couldn't even do a girl push up or dips. Pull ups were out of the picture for a long time. My muscle mass was not the same after having 13 lymph nodes removed. I still don't have much feeling in my armpit. It's hard to shave because it caves in and I have to be careful not to shave too deeply and cut myself. I really need to get laser hair removal for my underarm so I don't have to ever shave it again.

They removed all my breast tissue and fat to where, pretty much, nothing was left. Now I have a foreign device in me, a silicon implant, that is cold to the touch sometimes... which is crazy. I knew that I would get used to it; I didn't really have a choice. I would still push through and get my butt back in shape. Before I was diagnosed with breast cancer, I was probably in the best shape of my life physically... or so I thought. I used to workout with professional NFL players doing weight training and running. My body was the bomb back then but I didn't think so. I felt I was in good shape but I always wanted my stomach flatter and my abs banging. It's so funny how you are never satisfied with yourself. But looking back at pictures from the past, I shake my head. My body was amazing...even with all the shit I was putting in to it.

I remember telling my personal trainer I had breast cancer and how positive and supportive he was. He told the other guys and they got together and gave me some money to help when I was going to be out of work. I wasn't taking care of my inside as well as I was taking care of the outside. I was smoking and partying. I never had to buy drinks so I would get drunk almost every weekend. I couldn't turn down free drinks, right? I definitely had alcoholic tendencies. My Nanny, which is what I called my mom's mom, was an alcoholic. I could always smell the liquor coming out of her skin. My mom also had the same tendencies with drugs and alcohol, which she finally kicked in her 60s. I stopped smoking, drinking, and partying for a while.

My life was on a temporary hold. The guy I was seeing at the time was younger than me and that fizzled out. I didn't do much dating until I felt a little better about myself. In the back of my mind, I always thought, "Why would somebody want me when they could have a girl who had two good boobs and was not a cancer survivor?" I couldn't kick that thought for a while and retreated back to the old Erika who didn't give a shit about much, didn't think highly of myself, let others take advantage of me, and was needy and very lonely. I got into relationships with married men or guys who had multiple girlfriends. I didn't really look any different on the outside. I thought I could just pick up where I left off. I was still dealing with athletes, getting the same results. But this time, it didn't make me feel right. It was like I was trying to see if I could still get the guy even with what I had just gone through. I wouldn't tell the new guys that I just met that I had my breast removed because I had breast cancer. I would just make sure to keep my bra on and if they ever asked, I'd tell them why later. I knew most wouldn't ask. I was glad that they didn't because I knew I would be judged right away or they would want to see it. Men are so visual and it wasn't a pretty sight. They didn't really care. All they wanted was my cookie.

That high only lasted for me until the next one. I knew a lot of athletes, some just friends and some were obviously more. Of course, I always wanted the cute, sexy, bad boy. One of the teammates of the guy I was dealing with told me that my "boyfriend" was in the locker room telling everyone that I only had one real boob. I was the joke. The teammate told me to kick my boyfriend to the curb and hang out with him instead. He said he would give me $1000 just to hang out and keep him company. It's really important how you value yourself and your body. I had to continually remind myself that I had only lost my breast. Jesus had saved me. He had helped me with early detection and spared my life because he had bigger things planned for me on this journey we call life.

FREE ME 2 BE ME

Most of the guys were younger than me so their mentality was still very juvenile. This really allowed me to see what was wrong with me. I was still juvenile myself. I was still blocking my blessing with everything that I had just gone through. I still went back to the same life of destruction that would never give me what I wanted and what I really needed.

Now, I am working on becoming an advocate for breast cancer, working on being a better person, working on truly loving myself and being there to support my nephew and niece in the absence of my sister from their lives. My work will continue to be progressive, always evolving, finding and living in the grace of God, who has forgiven me for my sins. He has made me righteous for all His sacrifice on the cross.

I was back at work full time. My insurance took care of 80% of my surgeries so I would have some hospital bills coming in. Thank God they let me set up a payment plan. I got back to working out regularly to rebuild my chest muscle. The gym was my oasis. Pumping iron, spinning, Zumba, and just sweating it out was my therapy. When I go to the gym now, I go to locker number 100. It's just a mentality that I set for myself that I had gotten up and made it to the gym. Now I must give 100%. It's so funny because if there is already a lock on the locker, I cuss the lady out in my head. So, now I have to look for another locker maybe the 50 or just 99 because it's the closest to 100. It's crazy, but it works. I go in to class knowing I'm going to give everything I got because sometimes I don't know when my work schedule will allow me to get back in the gym. I do so much better in group classes having competition from the other ladies and guys because it keeps me motivated. I push myself harder. When I'm on the road, the hotel gym doesn't give me that same environment to push myself. But I remain positive. I just had to listen and apply what I preached because I did beat cancer. I was so blessed to have only lost my breast. It could have been a lot worse. I remember one time telling a flight attendant about my insecurities. I shared how I would make excuses for my lack of having a successful relationship or being enough because I only had one good boob. I also told him about the possibility of the cancer returning and the fear of men not wanting to date someone with one boob. He reminded me that I am more than my body parts and if I can't see that then I need to work on myself. He also reminded me that if any man couldn't see beyond that, I didn't need them in my life and that there was someone out there that would love me for the beautiful person I am. I really appreciated his words and have applied them in my daily life.

It is hard sometimes, but I am taking it one day at a time. I am loving myself, staying positive, knowing I am enough, and continuing to reach for and accomplish my goals. I am still a work in progress and still pushing forward until I reach that finish line. It really is a constant process through a lot of self-talk. When something doesn't go your way, you have to come up with a new plan of how to achieve that goal. You may have to try several ways, but just know that it will come together one piece at a time. Even if you take three steps forward and you have to take one step back, remember it's ok. Just get it together and keep taking those steps forward. Keep telling yourself, "I won't stop. I can't stop."

After learning to truly love myself and my new body, I was no longer afraid to tell my potential mates about my breast cancer and that I lost my breast. I am upfront. I don't try to hide my breast with my bra or keep my shirt on during sex. But I also take my time and date to see if the guy is even worthy of

FREE ME 2 BE ME

getting into my bed. The big change came after I got my mastectomy tattoo. It took so well to my scars. I didn't like looking at my scars so how could I think my mate would? We all know how visual males. But since I wasn't confident and comfortable with myself, how could I expect others to be? No one can say it was easy becoming the person you were meant to be. Step into it, take a chance, be brave and believe in yourself!

1. What is your favorite activity to do to stay active?

_____
_____
_____

2. What is one food you can't give up?

_____
_____
_____

3. Do you write out New Year's resolutions?

_____
_____
_____

4. Do you set goals for yourself?

_____
_____
_____

5. What makes you the happiest?

_____
_____
_____

> *"I'm an emotional creature. I'm giving, I'm loving. I'm often unappreciated, overlooked, and taken for granted. Not anymore! My eyes are wide open. Love yourself first… that's a must!"*

CHAPTER SIX

MENTOR, MENTOR WHERE FOR

Reassure: Put someone's mind at rest, encourage, cheer up, restore confidence.

During my research and visits to my doctors, I found a support group for young cancer survivors called Young Survival Coalition. YSC was for young women facing breast cancer together. Members had to be under 40 when you were first diagnosed. I started going to monthly networking meetings. We would have dinner and talk about how we were doing, how our treatments were going, and the next step in our process. We were just sharing our stories. We would also volunteer to welcome new survivors. It's not a club you really want to join but I'm so glad that I found them. It was great having other women to talk to who were going through the same thing. Although we all had different diagnoses, we all had breast cancer.

I started training to become a survivor navigator, helping other newly diagnosed survivors navigate their way through the process and giving guidance where needed. It was a great way to connect with other survivors and help them understand the process, cope with the emotional journey and manage their fears and anxiety. I assisted with social services and financial services to aid with their health needs. I also went to doctor appointments, invited them to meetings, and met for coffee just to talk. It helped me as much as it helped them.

It is really hard sometimes to be with your family and friends because they don't know what to say, or they feel they may say the wrong thing. Sometimes, they are more upset and emotional then you are and you have to calm them down. When someone is going through the same thing, it's easier to connect more openly and to tell them how you are really feeling. I would always tell family and friends to come hang out like we usually did. It helped me take my mind off of what was going on. I just wanted to laugh, go to the movies or dinner, or just sit and watch television. Their just being there with me meant a lot because some people didn't even show up for me. You don't always have to try to make anything better; just be there.

I really enjoyed helping other survivors for that reason. I hope I gave them some comfort or reassurance to take that next step in their process. I am very open about my cancer. You can ask me anything and I will gladly give my opinion. I will tell you how I feel about anything. I will show you what my boob looks like and let you touch it if you want. That is how open I am. Some survivors don't want to talk about it at all or only share with a few people. Just like breast cancer has many diagnoses, every woman or man handles their situation differently. There is no right or wrong way, just your way. I try to live my life not thinking about my cancer. I know I have to go to the doctor at least two times a year for my mammogram on my good breast and a breast MRI on the other breast. But in between those times, I live like cancer hasn't touched me. I'm not the nicest person when I do go to my appointments. I hate waiting and I hate getting my boob all smooshed up but I know it's what I need to do to take care of myself.

This past year was the worst. I have very dense breast and millions of cysts and they always seem to call me back in for a follow up because something looks suspicious. So last year was nothing new. I got the letter to make another appointment after having my mammogram. They saw something that they wanted to look at again. I scheduled my appointment to go in for an ultrasound with the possibility of getting a breast MRI, in the event they couldn't find what they were looking for with the ultrasound.

The one thing I love about going to my checkups is that the

hospital is literally across the street, so I can walk without having to look for parking or paying for it. So, I check in, put my robe on and wait to be called. My patience really sucks so I just talk to myself sometimes to relax. I'm getting better but I hate going to the doctor. They call me in to lay me down on the table, turn me sideways and apply that cool gel they use for the ultrasound. The tech runs the scope over my breast looking for masses they saw from my mammogram. She took a couple photos to show the doctor and stepped out of the room. I wait and wait for them to come back. Two female doctors come in and do the same thing the tech did and then tell me they want to do an MRI because it looks abnormal. So instead of getting, "Everything looks ok. Get dressed and go home," this time, they tell me I needed further tests.

They wipe all the gel off and tell me to come back in an hour for the test. They give me a voucher for the café. I always say a little prayer before my meals but that day, I asked God for some extra things… to continue to bless me, to continue to keep me healthy, and cancer free. So, I returned for my MRI. They give me a concentration that goes through my veins so they can see everything more clearly. I don't know what the tech did but when they set me up, I had to lay down face forward with my breast in the open space so they could be seen, and my feet elevated a little. I wanted ear plugs but the tech said the headphone would be on so I could hear the music. They roll you into a long cylinder with only my feet hanging out. It's cold and because I always freeze in the air conditioning, they have a blanket on me. It takes about 30 to 45 minutes. You can't move and the noise is horribly loud and annoying. The headphones did not help at all. I should have used ear plugs *and* headphone. Plus, I asked for R&B and she ended up playing some ghetto rap with bitch and hoes in it! While all this is going on, the

FREE ME 2 BE ME

concentration hits my veins. It's cold and it hits me like someone has punched me in the stomach. Now remember, I'm not supposed to move. I start getting the dry heaves. I thought I was going to throw up but I don't. Then my nose starts running. My arms are at my side so I can't wipe it or move. Snot just drips out of my nostrils.

When I look back on it, the whole situation is hilarious, but it wasn't funny while I was going through it. I just wanted to cry. All this was going on with the blasting of that horrendous noise in my ears. I felt like I was falling apart and couldn't wait for this test to be over. I knew I would have to retest. Argh! Finally it was over and they pulled me out. I told them everything that happened and they said maybe they could still get some good readings off of it. I was like I sure hope so because that was one of the worst experiences of my life. I told the tech about the headphones and how she played the wrong music. At that point, I was a big bitch. I couldn't wait to get home and get in my bed and curl up into a ball. It was the worst day almost ever! Weeks later, I received a letter from the doctors. I have to retest because they couldn't get a good reading. I had to go through all of it again! No! Well, hopefully minus all the stupid shit.

I set up my new appointment and arrived at the hospital. They set me up for my MRI and put the IV in so they could send the concentration through my veins. I told the tech about my last experience and she apologized and assured me this time would be different. I put the earplugs in and had the station on R&B. They set up my boobs in the machine and started the test. When they sent the concentration to my veins I didn't even feel. The noise wasn't so bad, but still annoying. I have to do this test at least once a year so I better get used to it. I came out of the cylinder and they told me they still see the same abnormality and will now need to do a biopsy. The doctors came in shortly after for the procedure. They numbed the area, inserted a needle into my breast, and removed some tissue to be tested. Then I had to wait for the results. I was a mess again. I knew that it was possible to get the cancer in my good breast but I had hoped it wouldn't come to that. That is why I opted not to have it removed when I was first diagnosed. I needed to have cancer in my other breast too before I would have it removed. I didn't have a family history of cancer so I never thought that I would have to worry about that. I hoped and prayed it was nothing. The area bruised for a couple days, but my breast must be very dense because I never have a problem with the pain when I get one.

I got a call that next week that everything was clear, no cancer, and the results were negative. They think that it was probably one of the many cysts that probably just burst and sent the particles around making it look suspect. Thank the Lord!! No more doctors for a while. I just need to eat right, get my workouts in, stay positive, and live as stress free as possible!

Six months went by fast. I had to set up an appointment for my breast MRI and since I was finally going to get an implant placed in my good boob instead of getting another lift, I needed to be checked. Everything went like clockwork, except for when the concentration hit my veins. I felt a thump in my belly and my mouth watered, but I held it together and got through the test. It came back all clear. Yay! I was planning to get my implant at the end of the summer so I could enjoy the sun, go to the beach and not worry about healing from a boob job.

I nixed the implant in my good boob and decided to wait until I had to replace the implant in my other boob. It has been 10 years, so I know that will happen soon. I haven't had any problems with it but that's what they tell you in the beginning. Since it's a silicone implant, that's the protocol. So, we will see how soon it happens. Then I can just have them both done at the same time. I have already had my mammogram for the year and got a letter that everything looked good so I have to set up my breast MRI soon. The dreaded breast MRI, but it must be done for my yearly visits to the hospital. One down, two to go!

I don't think people really understand that even though I'm cancer free, I still have to live my life hoping and praying that it doesn't come back. It's a scary reality. You try not to worry or stress yourself out every time something doesn't feel right or you get a sharp pain or a weird pull. You just can't live thinking or worrying if it will come back; you just have to live and stay positive. I try to put out positive posts on my social media because it really helps me as much as it may help someone else who might be following me.

I recently started working with another group, My Style Matters, as an advocate for breast cancer survivors and the disparities we face as a group with survivorship. In the Black community, 40% of women die from this disease compared to white women and are twice as likely to die if they are over 50. Being your own advocate is always best when discovering available options, as well as educating yourself and the communities you are a part of. With the increase in research for treatment of Black and Brown women, we can get a better understanding of how this disease grows in all women.

I went to Capitol Hill in Washington, D.C., last year to advocate for a survivorship care plan. I have been to several meetings to find out the new research and treatment plans that are in development. It's so crazy how things have changed. Sometimes I wonder if I had gotten my cancer now, how different my plan would be. I might even still have a viable nipple. My cancer was so low grade at Stage 1 that it probably wouldn't have even been removed. There's that would've, could've, should've again. But I'm glad the next lady will have better options and choices. I also went to my state capitol in Georgia to advocate for the disparity in the Black community and what is not covered by insurance. I would love to get more involved traveling around to different conferences and learn as much as I can to help the next survivor and to keep up on what I need to continue to do for my own survivorship.

Statistics show that 95% of cancer can be preventable through lifestyle changes. I have made changes in my life to prevent recurrence. My lifestyle includes working out regularly, trying to eat veggies and fruits daily, cutting fried food and foods filled with preservatives, drinking a lot of water, cutting sugary drinks out, and limiting my alcohol intake. Try to add one of these changes to your daily routine and add more as you go to have a better and healthier lifestyle. No one wants to be a part of this club but if you are, continue to fight the fight. Don't give up. Stay positive through the journey. You can survive this disease.

1. Do you have a mentor or someone you look up to? If yes, who?

_____
_____
_____

FREE ME 2 BE ME

2. Have you ever volunteered before? If yes, with who?

_____
_____
_____

3. Do you make a monthly budget? Do you usually stick to it?

_____
_____
_____

4. What is your guilty pleasure?

_____
_____
_____

5. What is your vice?

_____
_____
_____

> *"I have to stop wasting energy on things I can't control and things I can't change. I need to start listening to my body because it has all the answers. It knows what I need."*

ERIKA WEATHERS

CHAPTER SEVEN

PERCEPTION

Opinion: A personal view not necessarily based on fact or knowledge, the belief, judgement, impression or conviction of people in general.

ERIKA WEATHERS

I had been flying for about 15 years and I love my job, but I needed something more, something else to stimulate me... to challenge me. I went to Bartending School. My mom used to bartend and come home with a lot of cash. I knew I could make good money bartending. So, I got my certificate and tried to get a job. But since I didn't have any experience it was hard. Did I really want to be back in the club atmosphere getting hit on all the time? I think not. So I started taking golf lessons. It was fun and very challenging. I bought some clubs that still sit in my bedroom collecting dust. Golf is an expensive sport. You must have patience and someone to play with, so that wasn't going to work. Oh and did I say patience... which I'm always working on?

I had done some modeling when I lived in San Diego. I even did some extra work on the TV show Silk Stalkings. I had a couple featured extra spots and could have had a bigger role if I didn't screw it up, but I was too hungover from the previous night and missed my call time. I never got that shot again. I also did some extra work on the Jamie Foxx show because one of my friends knew Jamie. It was the Super Bowl episode. We were also featured in the Notorious music video with P Diddy and Lil Kim. It was like a movie with Tracey Morgan. It was fun, but we didn't get paid for it because my friend knew Diddy. Since I had dabbled in TV but never had training or an agent to get me real auditions, I started taking acting classes. Atlanta was starting to attract a lot more production companies. They were shooting movies and TV shows because of the great tax incentive that Georgia was offering. It was the perfect time to start training and get in the grind. They started calling Georgia the Hollywood of the South. Georgia is a right to work state so there are a lot of non-union gigs. Not being a part of SAG is good in the beginning of your career, but once you start booking better jobs

FREE ME 2 BE ME

you must join SAG, if it's a union project. At that point, you can no longer do non-union work or you could be fined.

I started at the Alliance Theater in 2010 and went to several different studios. I tried different methods like Meisner, Strasberg, improvisation and on-camera classes. It was very challenging and scary, but fun. I looked for auditions for indie projects on different websites. I still didn't have an agent so I had to find my own work. I went to auditions. Some were good, some were really bad, but it was a learning experience. I had to overcome my fears, build my confidence and just be myself. I'm still a work in progress.

I booked my first indie project in 2011, a web series called Idle Times. I played investigative reporter Brook Houston. I signed with my Agent Barbara Garvey with East Coast Talent in 2013. I got my first lead role on a re-enactment show with TV One called Fatal Attraction. I was the killer. It was a lot of fun. I had to drive to Knoxville, Tennessee, and check into hotel for the next three days. The experience was awesome. I got my makeup done, my wig fluffed, and had blood flicked in my face. I killed my boyfriend with a wrench and got paid to do it. I knew this was something I wanted to do so I had to continue to train and get better to book more jobs. I have since booked a training video for Well Fargo, a web ad for direct TV and other indie projects. Some are paid, some are not, but the experience is like free training. So, it's a win win. Sometimes, I would get some good footage out of it to add to my reel. I'm hoping to book a union SAG project, episodic or film real soon. From my mouth and fingers to God's ears!

I have had some great auditions but still haven't booked that big gig yet. Sometimes, I think I get so excited about being in a particular show that I put extra pressure on myself, especially when it's one of my favorite shows. I'm really good at self-sabotage. I must learn to get out of my head and just have FUN! I found an acting class that I really liked call P.A.N. - Premium Acting Network, which is run by Dwayne Boyd. It is mostly black actors. Every week there would be something different after our warm up. We'd warm up our voices and our bodies, then play games. Everyone would share if they had auditions, bookings or projects they were working on. We would then do improv, on-camera auditions, cold reads, or scene study and break up into groups, depending on how big the class was that evening.

During one of our classes, we had an exercise where the teacher asked us if we could talk to anyone dead or alive who would it be? We went to the front of the room and had a conversation with that person. I picked my ex-best friend because I hadn't really lost anyone close to me and the break up was still bothering me. As in any relationship, be it a boyfriend, girlfriend, parents, or siblings, when something goes unresolved or unanswered, it's bothersome. So, I acted like we were on the phone one last time and I asked her why she didn't want to be friends with me anymore? What was so bad about our last conversation? I was just expressing how I felt about her situation. Why do we always need or want to know what's in someone else's head? We want a conclusion, an ending, and when we don't get it, we have to make up our own ending. By the end of that exercise, I was crying and my teacher said that I had a breakthrough by getting up in front of the class and letting it all out, being vulnerable… just being. All my classmates were saying that I should try to reach out to her again. Some thought that she was my girlfriend "girlfriend", as in lover, because I was so upset. But I am strictly dickly. We just had a special connection over our 10-year friendship. We had some really good times and some really bad times. The fact that it ended the way it did really affected me. I don't know anyone who is good at any type of breakup.

I did reach out one more time but got nothing. This exercise really helped me to move on and has helped my acting. Once a year, we did a showcase and Dwayne invited casting directors and agents to check us out. There were so many opportunities to get an agent or to get on a casting director's radar. I only did one showcase but got some great feedback. I was contacted by a manager and got some audition invites from some of the casting directors. I still wasn't at the level to sign with a manager and I already had an agent. I still need to book my first 5 and under, which is a scene with five lines or less on a SAG project. I am still just booking indie projects, non-union commercials and some modeling gigs.

I took a marketing class to find out my essences, how I should be cast and what my type is. In class, we got up and tell a story about a place that we loved. For me, that was the beach. I love lying in the sun, hearing the waves roll in, walking on the beach when the sun is rising in the morning or setting in the evening. Oh how beautiful! My peaceful place! Another time was a story about my childhood when we had gotten in trouble. When I was younger at my grandparents' house in South Carolina, my twin, my cousin and I were playing in the tree and broke my uncle's mirror. We all said we didn't do it so we all got a whipping which was not fun. During this exercise, our classmates wrote something about us, their perception, a feeling that they got from us and handed it in. This was a new class so you didn't know anyone. From the answers, we were supposed to see if someone who knows nothing about us could really see the essence of who we were in just minutes. Some of the highlights on my list were: I was fake; a flirt; unbelievable; low energy; funny; matronly clear distinct voice; bitchy; caring; conceited; goofy; reflective; school teacher-ish; commanding of attention; and my favorite, your spirit is younger than your hairstyle. It is so crazy how people see you. The age range in the class was 20s-40s, and made up of different races and genders. I also sent surveys out to friends and family and had them remain anonymous, but I could figure out some of them. So, I received responses from a lot of people (boyfriends, girlfriends, classmates, co-workers) who have actually known me since I was a child. Here are some questions and answers narrowed down to the top 5...

Five adjectives you think describe me?

1. Strong

2. Adventurous

3. Beautiful

4. Loyal

5. Caring

Five things you think are my strengths?

1. Intelligent

2. Honesty

3. Planner

4. Independent

5. Ambitious

FREE ME 2 BE ME

Five things you think are my weaknesses?

1. Giving

2. Emotional

3. Too trusting

4. Patience

5. Vanity

If I were an animal, what would I be?

1. Cat family big and small - being cool, calm and collected, graceful, loner and deliberate movements

2. Dog females - loyal but can also be a bitch

3. Owl - you're wise

4. Fox - intelligent, sexy and sly

5. Gazelle - graceful and quick

If I were a piece of furniture what would I be?

1. Chaise lounger - laidback and relaxing

2. China Cabinet - It displays beautiful objects solid but fragile

3. Entertainment Center - people like to gather around it and be entertained

4. Couch - comfortable

5. Dining room table - intimate, stylish and inviting

If I were a 3-year-old now, what would I get in trouble for

most?

1. Talking back

2. Disappearing

3. Wanting what I ask for now

4. Poking lips out and rolling eyes

5. Too active

Name something about me that you think would surprise people?

1. Used to burp like a hippo

2. Have a twin

3. Nickname Ricki

4. Look unapproachable but really friendly

5. Jumped out of a plane 2 times

What word or phrase would you use to describe me in a romantic relationship?

1. Loving

2. Emotionally immature

3. Powerful

4. Intoxicating

5. Committed

This was very insightful. After looking at it again after five years,

FREE ME 2 BE ME

it's even more so. My own perception of how I view myself has changed. I narrowed it down to some of the things in common from the people who knew me to the people who didn't. I compiled some of the words that stuck out from the surveys and notes. My teacher then came up with six essences that were spot on.

1. Self-contained

2. Shaking on the inside, fearless on the outside

3. Rainbow on a sunny day!

4. Champagne is always appropriate!

5. Boldly lighting the path in front of you.

6. Secret romantic

Develop your own list of 5 questions to ask friends and family to help you and see what you come up with. Have fun with it!

My whole perspective is different. The way I watch movies and television is so different. I'm paying more attention to the actor and the way he/she moves me or not. I try to see all the Oscar-nominated films and see if I can pick the winners. I can see the great acting, the good acting and the bad acting. I can see how actors evolve over their careers. Most get better along the way.

I met a friend of a friend who was into fitness modeling. She used to be one of the girls working out behind the fitness pro. She had a lot of connections. She got divorced and moved to Los Angeles. After my divorce, I started hanging out more with her and some of her other friends going to parties. Her birthday is the day after mine but she would play like she forgot my birthday so she could celebrate hers. That should have told me something right there, but if you know me, you know that I love to celebrate my birthday, especially the milestone ones. I almost wonder why I hung around her sometimes. I now think that the prettier the girls were around her, the better. That was until she got what she wanted... a rich famous husband. We had great times back then hanging out in Los Angeles, going to parties, going to the beaches in Miami, Super Bowls, and all-star games. I met a lot of people but I wish I had made better connections. Back when I was younger, I was never into a lot of makeup. I was naturally pretty. I wasn't even plucking my eyebrows. I was like one of these girl you could fix up with makeup. I was the project girl with these girls so just imagine what that looked like... the Mexican, the Thai and black, the white and black mix, the white girl and I was the black and Italian. We were a pretty hot ass group. Out of the 5, 3 of us were Leos. I got invited to the baby shower but not the wedding. I think it was small since both had been married before. Her new husband was one of Halle Berry's ex-husbands. I was the girl who never had her nails done, didn't care about a boob job and I didn't need a weave. I was the cute sporty one and that is still me today. I'll get my nails and hair done on occasion but I still don't wear makeup, unless I'm hanging with my girlfriends. I'm still single so I don't even worry about shaving on a consistent basis or tweezing my eyebrows. Boyfriends and husbands are a lot of work. The other girls had enhancements and were more glamorous. She was also the same friend who said that now I can get a boob job because I got breast cancer. She was so superficial. She was the kind of girl who went to bed with makeup on. She could be so sweet, then talk about you behind your back in a minute.

None of my Leo girlfriends were ever around for long. We all had too much fire. We were leaders, bossy, and gregarious. Someone had to give up their power or the friendship would dissolve. It's funny. My stepmom and older sister are both Leos and at this point in my life, I don't have a relationship with either. I did enjoy the times we spent together. We were hanging out with entertainers, actors and athletes. They were some of the biggest names in the game at the time. I went to the premiere of Janet Jackson's movie Poetic Justice and met Tupac and some other stars. I got a glimpse of Janet but didn't meet her. I used to love that Janet album. It was one of my favorites. Her abs were on fire. I kept a picture in one of my journals for inspiration. I think that I still have it and I'm still obsessed with my abs. I got to see her in concert when she did the velvet rope tour. She is such a great dancer and performer.

When you're married to a professional football player, you get to meet a lot of athletes. Some were the most famous in their sports, some just friends and others were more than friends. I look back at where some of the careers of some of the greatest players in the NFL, NBA, and MLB have gone. It's crazy how so many of the guys I knew then, now have jobs as commentators. I used to only date athletes. I was so in the know about most sports. I used to watch ESPN 24/7 like a lot of the athletes. I love the games, especially football and basketball. My favorite commentator was Stuart Scott. He had this saying, "Cool as the other side of the pillow." He passed from cancer. When I lived on the west coast during football season, I could watch football all day long. The first game came on at 10 a.m., then another at 1 p.m., and 5 p.m. I used to love to play in a football pool where you picked straight up games with no points and no fantasy football. It made the game more fun to watch. I never looked at myself as a groupie. I just loved sports and some of the men that played them. I mean I was considered a dime piece, or wifey material. If only I had respected myself enough to not play games after my divorce. If only I had been smart enough to realize it's really not just about sex. Yes, for some it is, but a lot of men want a good girl. They want someone who hasn't been with a lot of athletes or entertainers. But I fell into my old destructive ways and found some new party girls to do it with. I was happy being single... or so I thought.

Most of the big superstars were cheaters with multiple girlfriends or even married. They didn't care because if you didn't do it, another girl would come around and give them what they wanted. I finally stopped dating athletes when the last guy I was with turned out to be the same old liar. I thought he was different until his friend told me he was engaged. He lied to me, saying he didn't think he was going to like me so much. He told me that he used to watch me when I was out with my girlfriends and that I seemed to be cool.

I recently connected with him accidentally. He was divorced and had two kids. We met for lunch. It was so good to see him. I had been single for almost three years, since ending a relationship. I have dated a little, but I stopped online dating and was concentrating on me. So, it was a welcomed surprise. I think it was a reminder to never go back to relationships that were based on lies. Men who have tons of money grow older but all don't grow up. He seemed like he was still doing the same things as before. He was dating several women, lying and cheating, and still thinking he could do whatever he wanted just because. I couldn't and wouldn't go back to a relationship like that because it would be a situation not a relationship. I had grown, matured, and realized I needed and wanted more from a relationship. I'm not sharing with anyone else; I would rather be all by myself.

FREE ME 2 BE ME

2020... What a year! I thought it was going to be a year full of travel. I would have my five weeks of vacation back, my seniority back, and a raise after contract negotiations. I started the New Year in Panama City, Panama, with my girlfriends. We celebrated 2020 out of the country for the first time. We had a great time. The city was beautiful and very metropolitan. I wasn't expecting that. In February, I went to Kona, Hawaii, with my girlfriends and the family I lived with during my senior year. We had a late celebration for our 50th birthdays. Jenny was turning 50 that May. Hawaii is one of my favorite vacation spots. It never disappoints me. I have been to Oahu three times so I was glad to go to another island. I still need to go to Maui. In March, I had an Airbnb set up for Amsterdam. My girlfriend was going to Paris for her 50th and she was going to take a train to Amsterdam to hang out for a couple of days. I wanted to go to the red light district, smoke some weed or eat some edibles, maybe go to a porn show, visit the museum and go to the Heineken plant. I was so excited. It was going to be a busy March. I had a conference the first weekend with the Young Survivor Coalition. I was going to be a moderator for a couple of the events and go to the Bill Maher Show. I finally got tickets to go and my sister was going to go with me. I was going to plan a trip each month of the year and then COVID-19 hit. The world started shutting down that first weekend in March. Our flight schedules started tanking in April, May, June, and July. I had taken time off without pay and went on unemployment because of the Care Act. The airlines couldn't furlough anyone until the end of September, unless it was extended. And as we had all experienced, congress hasn't done a damn thing but fight back and forth with each other. I went back to work in August with a limited schedule and was placed on reserve for the month of September. We had all hoped that the virus would have been contained in three months, then maybe six months. Concerns were that fall and winter may be worse.

Our flying schedule with United wasn't confirmed and we found out that United was deciding on which regional airline they were going to keep. Both were operating the 145 aircraft, 50 seater and we lost out to CommutAir because their operational costs were cheaper and they had less employees. So after flying with ASA/ExpressJet for 23 years, my career was coming to an end. I had gambled and stayed with the company through the ups and down hoping and praying I would make it 25 years to get my free flying benefits. I knew my shot with Delta was out the window, but when United bought us, and I had flown under their umbrella for a year and met the parameters of 20 years and 45 years, I, at least, thought that even though I was furloughed that I would be eligible for my flight benefits. We were so optimistic but on the last day, we were told United wouldn't be honoring the deal. Just like Delta, neither gave a shit about loyalty. It wouldn't even cost them a thing and all seats are stand-by, but it was still a no. All they care about is their bottom line.

I worked my last flight September 2, 2020, and then furloughed on September 30, 2020. I really can't see myself flying again especially for the majors because I would have to start over from the bottom, with no seniority and 1st flight attendant pay. I would maybe fly for a charter but realistically I think my flight attendant career is over. I'm 51 and the time spent at home has been very enjoyable. I don't miss the commute, my crash pad, or the overnights. I just miss being able to fly free and go anywhere at the last minute. But I wouldn't be going anywhere with what is going on in the world right now anyway. I think it has slowed everyone down so we can realize what is important... and that is to figure out what we really want out of life, instead of continuing in the rat race that we get trapped in. It's easier to keep doing what is comfortable, what you know is paying the bills, then to take a risk. I tell everyone that my job as a flight attendant was like a bad relationship you can't get out of because you don't want to be alone or because it's not *that* bad. But when you're not given the option and the boyfriend breaks up with you, everything goes out the window and it's over. Now, I have to do what is best for me to really try and find my true love, something that will satisfy my mind, my body and my soul. I know I want to travel the world. I know I want to keep my body in shape and stay cancer free. I know I want my creative juices flowing with my acting, writing, drawing, and something that stimulates me. I know I don't want a 9-5 so I have to figure it out and I will.

> *"I sit in front of the mirror, I notice my flaws, my scars, and my imperfections... They are mine. They are part of my story. I celebrate them because they are what make me uniquely me! As the years go by, and the older I get, I realize the imperfections make me more interesting. They make me unique, so I embrace them because they are what makes me truly beautiful."*

ERIKA WEATHERS

CHAPTER EIGHT

IT'S BACK

Insecure: Not firmly fixed or attached, lacking confidence, anxious

I stopped taking Tamoxifen after two years. I didn't like the way I felt when I was on it. Another two years passed and I was going in for my regular checkups, doing monthly breast exams, getting yearly mammograms, and seeing my oncologist. I was eating healthy. I was not smoking. I was back on a good workout routine. I had completed all my reconstructive surgery and was happy with my results. I was feeling good. That was until I started noticing a growth on my breast very close to my reconstructed nipple. Yes, the growth was growing on the same breast I had my mastectomy on. Usually five years is the mark we cancer survivors strive for. That gives us a chance of our cancer not recurring and the percentage of the cancer coming back drops. I was one year short. I didn't go back to see my doctor until after the holidays. I wanted to enjoy the season and the rest of the year. I made an appointment to see my doctor and he wanted me to get it biopsied. It turned out to be what he thought... the same cancer I had been diagnosed with the 1st time was back. My doctor said sometimes the cancer is still breathing when they cut it out so some of the cells may be left behind. When I was closed back up, it started growing again. It's not very common but it does happen. He said that they probably should have radiated me the first time just to make sure it was dead.

So, that is what we did the second time around. I had to reschedule my surgery and pretty much have everything done all over again. I kind of knew what to expect with my surgery. I didn't know how the radiation was going to be, but I thought I would be able to work through it. I worked a nap line. I wouldn't have to be to work until 7 or 8 p.m. and I would get off the next morning about 8 or 9 a.m. I would go home and walk across the street for my treatments at 11 a.m. Yes, I lived that close to my hospital... Emory Crawford. It actually worked out pretty well.

FREE ME 2 BE ME

First, they cut the cancer out again, removed my implant, and put tissue expander back in so that the radiation wouldn't melt my implant.

I healed from surgery and started my 36 radiation treatments. They were Monday-Friday at 11 a.m. for almost two months. My treatment was localized to my breast area, so it limited effects to my lungs and heart. It didn't burn too much. I had some fatigue towards the end of treatment but for the most part, it wasn't so bad because I was young and in pretty good health for being a cancer patient. I also applied emu oil to protect my skin because the radiation really does affect the way the skin heals. After re-stretching my expander with the injections, my implant was replaced in about six months. It took almost a year for the whole procedure of getting my new implant before the Christmas holiday. I decided not to redo the tattoo this time. I still had some of the tattoo leftover, plus the new scar from when they removed the cancer was darker and not as smooth because the skin had been radiated. I didn't feel like going through another surgery to make a nipple again so I opted to leave the scar. I thought maybe I could get a 3D tattoo or a mastectomy tattoo down the line because I knew I really didn't want to look at my scar every day. But I was fine for the time being.

It was a long 2008, but I was cancer free again. I went back on Tamoxifen for 3 years in order to have it in my system for the full 5 years as it was prescribed. Taking the Tamoxifen this time felt like I was taking a water pill. I was still getting my period with no bad side effects. It was crazy but I wasn't complaining.

I healed after my surgery. I was still working with YSC going to meetings and volunteering as a navigator. I had gotten back into the gym, started taking spin class and loved it. It was such a great cardio class that I would be drenched afterward. It wasn't good if I wanted to wear my hair straight, but I loved it and had my own shoes.

In 2009, YSC in Atlanta was having its first tour de pink. This was a bike ride to raise money for young women with cancer. I decided to participate. I put up flyers at work, sent out Facebook posts and was the second highest survivor to raise money. I raised almost $2,000.00 and I won a gift package with workout gear from Lucy. It was so great. I had borrowed a bike from a friend and clocked 18 miles on the ride. Those spin classes were great training. It was great fun and a great turnout for the first event. After that, I turned into a fitness fanatic. One of my girlfriends asked me to run a half marathon with her in San Diego. I was back on my fitness routine and started training with the Atlanta track club because I wasn't really a runner. I used to be a sprinter in high school, but even back then when we practiced, I never wanted to run long distance. I would say, "I'm a sprinter. Why do I need to run long distance?" If I had only realized how that would have made me a better conditioned and faster runner. But I didn't care about that then. I was too busy partying, not worrying about getting better. If only I had known then what I know now, I could have beaten that girl at states!

The track club was training for the Peachtree Road Race. So the coach gave me a training plan for my half marathon. I would run with them and then do some training on my own. The longest run I got in before the race was 9 miles so I felt pretty confident that I would be able to do the full 13.1 miles. The day of the race in June 2010, the weather was perfect. But what else would you expect from San Diego. I still loved this city even though I hadn't been back in years. We started at Jack Murphy Stadium and ended at Sea World. I ran my own race. My girlfriend and I started off together, then she took off. I had to keep my pace and not overexert myself. I finished in about 2:36. When I crossed the finish line, I almost hyperventilated. It was such a proud moment for me. I had set a goal and I accomplished it! After the race, we got in the hot tub. My body was feeling it. I could hardly walk. I ordered a cheeseburger, fries and a corona. I was in heaven.

In 2011, I signed up for the lottery for the Peachtree Road Race and got in the first time. It's a big event so that's the only way to get in, unless you are sponsored by one of the sponsors. The race is 10k, which is 6.2 miles and I finished in about 45 minutes. That cardiac hill really is no joke. At the end of 2011, I did a sprint triathlon with one of the flight attendants. This is considered a half triathlon, which consists of a 5k run, a 12-mile bike ride, and a 400-meter swim. I trained at my gym in the pool. That was probably the hardest part. I know how to swim, but not for a long period of time. Thank God this event was in a pool and not in a lake or the ocean. It was being held in October, so the water would have been pretty cold.

I also did the Merrell Down & Dirty Obstacle Mud Run with my sister. It was a 5k obstacle course. I did that race the next two years with my niece. It was a fun race. We were covered in mud by the end of it and had to hose off. I also ran the Spartan race which was also a 5k obstacle course but much more challenging. I did that with several of my girlfriends. I was always up for a challenge, something new and exciting.

In 2012, I did the YSC tour de pink again but just raised enough money to participate. I had stopped asking for donations for the cause. I felt like I was always asking every year for donations for something I was doing with breast cancer. I just couldn't do it anymore. I was getting discouraged with all the money that wasn't going to the survivors or how little of it was actually going to research. I'm so glad that I experienced all of these race events, but I won't be running a half marathon again, let alone a full marathon. If I had to run 5 straight hours, I don't know what I would do. It's not for me. I'll just stick to the bicycle and shorter runs. I was still into my spin classes. That was one of my favorite workouts when I was training for the different races. The music was such a motivating factor for me. But it was hard to find a teacher who played great music, and when I did, they didn't stay around long enough.

The craze for spin was ridiculous. You had to sign in at the desk to get a bike. People started showing up early just to get a bike with their favorite teacher. Nowadays, the classes aren't full at all. I do better in my workouts in groups because I like the motivation from the other people. I kind of feed off of them because I don't want to be the one stopping first or finishing last. It's all about competition. When I work out by myself, I feel like it's just an ok workout. I know I don't push myself hard but at least I get a sweat in and burn some calories. I really need to do better at pushing myself and not have to rely on others for motivation.

When I turned 50, my fitness goals were to do five 5k races, one for every decade that I have been on this planet. The first one I ran was in February, the morning of the Super Bowl Sunday. It was in Atlanta and it was pretty cold. I ran with my girlfriend Evelyn, who is a marathoner. The last one ended in the Mercedes Dome on the field which was pretty cool. I ran that one with my girlfriend Maria and her daughter.

FREE ME 2 BE ME

This year, my fitness goal is to run in a track meet for master's people over 50. I want to get back into my sprinting and find a master's track meet I can get involved with. I would like to run the 50- and 100-yard dash and possibly a 4x4 relay, if my speed is good enough. This goal is still in the works.

I've always said I was going to cut my hair short when I became pregnant, but that never happened. But when my company announced that they were sponsoring a locks for love event, I signed up. This was another way to give back to other cancer survivors by using my hair so that a child could have a wig made. I had my hair cut into a mushroom, but I didn't like it so I found someone who specialized in short cuts and told them to give me the Halle Berry cut. I loved it. I didn't know how I would look after having long hair pretty much my whole life but the upkeep was too much. I'm used to pulling my hair back and wearing it curly, but I had to go to the salon more regularly because I was natural and my hair didn't want to lay down. I worked with it and eventually let it grow back through the awkward stages. At least I found out what my hair looked like in all stages. When my hair grew back again, I did the locks of love one more time. I learned that they were selling some of the wigs and not giving them away for free. I hope several cancer patients enjoyed their wig and that it puts a smile on their faces.

1. What do you absolutely love about yourself?

_____
_____
_____

2. What one thing about yourself needs a lot of work?

_____
_____
_____

3. What one thing do you wish that you could change about yourself?

_____
_____
_____

4. How happy are you about what you do for a living? Would you change careers if you could?

_____
_____
_____

5. What one thing makes you the happiest?

_____
_____
_____

> *"Invest in yourself. Do what you have to do. Take care of yourself and be at peace with your decisions. There is only one you. Protect your heart, respect your body and listen to your intuition. All the answers are right there in front of you. You just need to pay attention."*

CHAPTER NINE

TAKE ADVANTAGE OF WHATEVER

Use: The privilege or benefit of using something or someone, exploit unfairly, the power of control.

Do you ever look back on your life and wonder if you took the right door, the right train, or picked the right state? One different decision in your life could have drastically changed the whole outlook of how your life would have ended up. Regret? Satisfied?

I wouldn't be who I am today if I took that other door. Yes, I would have probably had a child and yes, that's one of the biggest regrets in my life. But obviously that wasn't in the plan. Maybe having my nieces and nephews in my life is enough. It has to be enough. That's it! I am enough. No looking back over my shoulder on what could have been, wishing I had better family relationships, a successful marriage, more money, or that I never got cancer. God already had my plan mapped out.

I wake up every day and thank the Lord for blessing me. I'm not very religious; I have gone to church over the years but I have never read the whole bible even though I have tried to make it a priority over the years. I speak to God every day. I believe I'm more spiritual when I do go to church. I love the atmosphere and I'm still trying to find a church home that feels most inviting to me. I seem to cry freely just listening to the word and I'm always drawn to come down and join the church but I don't. My cousin told me that I'm purging, that I have a broken heart and instead of mending it, I brush things off my shoulders, try to be strong and keep it moving. It makes sense, but I don't know how to fix it. Hopefully I am a step closer to learning how to do that, how to deal with my issues straight on and stop shuffling them to the side. I have never spoken to anyone professionally about it but maybe I should. Maybe this book is my therapy.

I now believe that my broken heart is from my father. Our

relationship over the years has had some ups and downs. It's been a rollercoaster ride with him and my stepmother. They are a package deal. At the end of the day, I have never gotten the love I really needed from him. He has never really stepped up for me in the way I needed him to. It had always been my stepmother who would make the decisions whether to help us out or buy us things, or to make kind gestures or not. There was a time that I thought I could count on him but it never happened.

When I was diagnosed with cancer, I knew he would come visit me after my surgery while I was out of work and recovering. My mom, my sisters, and my girlfriends all came, but my stepmother said, "Oh, you have your mother. You don't need your dad to come." And he let that be his answer. He likes to always say, "Do the right thing," but I don't think he has always done the right thing. It was just another disappointment, another chip at my heart. They did send some money to help with my bills while I was out on medical leave, but all I wanted was for him to come be by my side, even if it was only for a day. Everything isn't always about money. Having real genuine loving relationships is what life is really about, but so hard to find.

As I was beginning to write my book, I had a falling out with my dad and stepmom just before the Christmas holiday. I finally made it home to New York for Christmas. I hadn't been there for years and didn't even see or speak to them over something I posted on Facebook. Yes, I know Facebook is responsible for many family feuds, but this one was very petty. I didn't have any motive behind posting a picture of myself and my twin brother. It was just blown out of proportion and neither one of us has reached out to the other. I have since tried to call my dad but I've received no answer or returned call. I asked my older brother if they ask about me because when they wouldn't talk to my sister they got updates from me about what she was doing now. My brother told me that they hadn't asked about me and that they only hear about when I visit my brother Chris or sister Tara or if they are looking at my Facebook page. I know I'm blocked from their pages but they can probably still see mine because I didn't block anyone. My brother told me that my father said that I disrespected him, which is why he wasn't talking to me and didn't want to add any more stress to my stepmother's life. He has no concern about my stress level. But it's all good. It makes me sad but I can't fret about it.

The relationship has always been stressful for me. It should have been done years ago. I know they won't be happy about me writing a book about my life, my family, or about me showing pictures of my half-naked body. But this is MY story. All I have ever wanted was my parents to be proud of me for the woman that I have become, to have a stress-free, carefree, loving, respectful, meaningful relationship with my mom, my dad, my stepmother, and all of my siblings. But we don't always get what we want. I get that. I have tried and tried again but I have given up.

The only constant in my life is my mom. She has really stepped up. Years ago, she quit drugs and only drinks on special occasions, if at all. I speak to her almost every day. I won a $1,000 gift card for Apple at one of my conferences for breast cancer and bought her and myself an IPad. Now we FaceTime every day. It's been great and she is doing great in her 70s. She is always here for me when I need her. I have forgiven her years ago for the past. We have moved on and have a great loving and carefree relationship. I can say anything I want and not have to feel like I said it the wrong way or worry about it being misinterpreted. We started traveling years ago. She can fly for free as well so we plan a trip once a year together. We went to Italy first since my mom is half Italian and I am a quarter. We flew to Rome, went to all the attractions, took a bus ride to Naples, a boat ride to Capri and Sorrento, and a train ride to Venice. We had five days. It was planes, trains, buses and boats. Italy is such a beautiful country. We got to see a lot. We didn't make it to Florence to see the leaning tower of Pisa but it was still a great trip.

Aruba was next. It was so beautiful with very tranquil beaches and water. When we went, the natural beach was still standing. I have a picture of us on it. It was made out of sand and had been standing for years until a hurricane came and destroyed it. That island was only six miles by nine miles. I would love to go back.

The first time I went to Hawaii was with my mom. We went to Oahu and stayed in Waikiki. We could walk to the beach from our room. We went to a luau on the dole plantation. I fell in love with the sacred landscapes, the breathtaking views, and rainbows almost daily from the tropical rainstorms. I don't really like to revisit a location because there are so many new spots to explore but Hawaii is my magical place.

We picked Costa Rica on the Liberia side next. We stayed at a new hotel. It was so new that it wasn't fully staffed and not a lot of guests were there. This was the first time I saw black beaches. We went zip lining for the first time. My mom even did it. She really enjoyed it and said that the harness felt great on her back. They used a horse to get her through the forest. We went to the hot springs and the mud baths. It was so ooey and gooey. The mud was thick and it felt so go on our bodies. We let it dry and then rinsed it off in the hot springs.

In Jamaica, I went water skiing for my second time while my mom sat in the boat. My first time parasailing was there as well. We took cruises to Grand Cayman and visited Hell, a group of short, black, limestone formations located there.

In Honduras, I went swimming with the dolphins. In Grand Turks, we went snorkeling. My mom tried but her feet kept cramping from the flippers. It was beautiful. We went to Las Vegas, took a bus to the Hoover Dam, and then on to the Grand Canyon, where I walked out on the ledge to view the canyon. We flew to Seattle, went to the space needle, and then on to San Francisco to visit the Golden Gate Bridge and the Fisherman's Wharf. All the tourist spots were so cool. My mom doesn't get around like she used to and it's so hard to get seats on the plane. It's just too much for her now. I'm just glad I had the chance to experience those adventures with her.

I knew I had to forgive my father for not being the man I needed, and the dad I had always wished for him to be. I knew he probably didn't get what he needed from his parents/my grandparents. I just wish things were different. We aren't getting any younger and there is so much more living to do. I have so many more chapters to write that I want my family to be a part of. I did reach out to him on Father's Day because of a guy I was dating. He had a great relationship with his daughters and told me to call my dad so I thought about it and picked up the phone. He didn't answer but I left a message. I never got a call back. I tried. I reached out but now I'm done.

My sisters and brothers have always had me wondering if I hadn't kept in contact or visited them over the years would we even have a relationship. With me being a flight attendant, who can fly for free when seats are available, it's easier for me to visit or get an overnight in Detroit on occasions to have lunch, dinner or drinks with my twin brother. He has probably been to Atlanta three times... for my wedding and several times for our birthday. The last was on our 50th.

Chris really isn't good with keeping in touch with anyone in the family, except my dad and stepmom. He is always on their side when things go down. He doesn't like confrontation and just goes with the flow. He usually calls me on our birthday but we don't talk on a regular basis and I'm usually the one who calls. I usually go to California every December, right before the Christmas holiday, and help my stepsister put up her Christmas tree and decorate. I also help wrap presents.

Since I didn't have kids or a partner to always share the holidays with, that was my holiday cheer. We have been doing it for years. It has turned into a tradition. I love my stepsister and I wish I had a similar relationship with her mother because it makes it hard to not talk about the elephant in the room. When I'm not communicating with my dad and stepmom, my stepsister doesn't like to get involved. She says, "Sorry you have to deal with that." I told my stepsister that if she doesn't come to Atlanta, I'm not coming back to Los Angeles. So, she came with my nephew, Diego, for a couple days. Diego was going to Argentina for the summer and she had to get him on the plane out of Atlanta. It worked out perfectly. She was supposed to come this year but waited too long to get the tickets and the prices were crazy. I don't know what's going to happen this Christmas.

My older brother lives in New York close to both my mom, my dad and stepmom. He usually picks me up when I come to town. We talk on occasion and he's said over the years that he would come visit but hasn't been here in years. My oldest sister lives here in Atlanta but the relationship is nonexistent. We both love each other, but just don't like each other.

I remember when I went to live with her and her family in San Diego. I was so grateful for the opportunity she offered me to start my life. So when she needed to stay with me when she came to Atlanta for a new job, I was open to her staying with me until she got on her feet. I live in a one bedroom loft that is 744 square feet with no door on the bedroom. It's great for one person or a couple, but not ideal for a roommate. I was working three or four day trips at the time, so she got to enjoy my place more than me. I remember coming home one day and she was wearing a pair of my sneakers. She didn't ask if she could wear them and made me feel like I shouldn't even question her because I wasn't wearing them. It was crazy because they were at the top of my closet so that let me know she was going through my shit. She had to take the ladder out to get to the top and just assumed that I wasn't using them, so she would.

It had been about three months since the job she came to Atlanta for had been rescinded, because the paperwork wasn't filled out probably. She ended up staying with me longer until she found another job. It seemed like everything she did got on my nerves. I couldn't wait to go to work but also hated leaving thinking about what she was getting into while I was gone. I helped her get a job with one of my friends working security. She screwed up that friendship when she took an insurance check for damage to one of the vehicles and deposited it into her account instead of the business's account. My friend took her to court for the money and they ended up on the Judge Mathis TV show. She lost the case, of course, because she owed him the money. She countersued saying that he owed her money and that's why she took the check. She felt that this was the only way she would get it back. She looked so crazy on the show, trying to act like she did nothing wrong.

I'm kind of an auntie mom to her two kids who also live here in Atlanta. My lil Tweety Bird Brittany and Michelin baby Branden are both in their 30s. I have been in their lives on and off for years until they both ended up in Atlanta. Branden came here after he graduated college and Brittany moved here after having Jaylen to start her life after leaving college. I have tried to be there for them since their mother is pretty much nonexistent in their lives as well. She pops in and out depending on if she needs something. I could never understand her outlook on life, never accepting responsibility for the things that have gone wrong in her life. It was always someone else's fault as to why she got fired. She would pick a guy over having a relationship with her children. She could never really get it together. It is really a sad story but you can't help people who really don't want it. I just pray she is ok and finds happiness in her life.

As I sit here thinking about my father and stepmother, I really do believe that everything happens for a reason. We have not communicated since December 2017. It's funny the conversation that turned into an argument was between myself and my father. My stepmother never spoke on the phone that day but I know she was listening the whole time. They are always on the phone together and usually it's her doing all the talking. It was like he was provoking me and proving himself to her, like I was meddling again. I have gone over that conversation in my mind many times since that day. I was in Omaha waiting on a flight so I could start my work day. I was going to call them about my plans of coming home that

Christmas and maybe getting together for dinner. I had broken up with my boyfriend that summer so I wouldn't be in North Carolina that Christmas. I was going to go home for a long overdue visit so I thought it was going to be a good conversation.

During that conversation, my father said, "You don't have a boyfriend anymore so you have to start meddling with your brother again." You know when you're lost for words and become fearful of what you really want to say? Well, if he thinks I was disrespectful, then I know my tone changed pretty quickly because I was being accused of doing something intentionally and that was not the case. My stepmother and I have had disagreements over the years and have stopped talking for months, just never years. It's very disheartening the way the whole situation transpired. The last time I tried to reach out, it didn't happen. I have had several male friends in my life that have been nudging me to pick up the phone and call. I am glad I tried but I'm also glad he didn't answer. I know that doesn't make sense but it does to me. I feel like my life has been less stressful. I haven't had to worry about talking to them worrying if it was going to be a good or bad call. It was really a very toxic, dysfunctional relationship. I am going to stop giving so much of myself to all of the relationships I have with family, friends, and boyfriends.

Until I get married again, the only one that gets all of me is my mom. Yes, I will lose more family members, more girlfriends and plenty more boyfriends, but I am ok with that because my circle will be really small and the people remaining in that circle will be my ride or die. They will love me for me, regardless of what comes out of my mouth. They won't just love me for what I can do for them but because they care about me and care about how I am doing. I saw this quote that I just loved. It said, "Everyone should not have the same type of access to you." Think about it. It's so true. #learning

2017 was really a bad year for me. I broke up with my boyfriend, William. He was a Marine living in Jacksonville, North Carolina. The relationship was showing a lot of cracks after about a year because it was a long-distance relationship and it seemed I was the one making the most effort. Every time I wanted him to come to Atlanta, something would happen and he couldn't make it. He missed a film premiere for one of my indie films where I won best actress. He missed my nephew's wedding, a gala that was honoring my agent and several concerts I had planned. It was almost always the same excuses. It was crumbling. He didn't look at me the same way he used to. I felt like the honeymoon was over. When we first got together, it was like he was grooming me to be his wife. He wanted me to learn Marine rankings and understand his world. He took me to a retirement ceremony so when he retired I would know what to do. I went to a GI Jane event that they had for the women to experience what the Marines go through. It was pretty cool. I had all this gear on. I was shooting targets with a rifle doing all different kinds of drills. We went to the gun range so I could learn how to shoot. I really thought that I had come full circle ending up with a Marine. I thought he was going to be my husband.

The distance was a big factor because I was only there on weekends, sometimes during the week, but not enough for us to get into a routine of really learning from each other and for me to be comfortable with being able to call him my best friend. I started thinking he was cheating but he denied that saying he's not good at cheating so he doesn't do it. My intuition was telling me otherwise. When my mom finally came to town to meet his parents, it was so uncomfortable. He wasn't warm or inviting. He even said that I was just a rental, but said he was just joking. Of course, I didn't take that as a joke and we broke up after that weekend. Then we ended up getting back together a month later and that was when I bought my motorcycle hoping that would keep up together. It did for a couple more months, till it was over again, and I had to have him bring my motorcycle to Atlanta.

So, when my father used that relationship as a dig, it was very hurtful. The break up was in July. I was at least hoping to get to my birthday so I could get one more gift. We didn't make it. He knew what he was doing. You have to see the humor in every situation. The break up with my father and stepmother was about five months later right before Christmas. I never realized that almost four years later that relationship would be nonexistent and that it would all be blamed on me. Two men that I loved, one for a lifetime, the other for several seasons, but both very devastating. It was especially devastating losing my father's relationship. I have been starving for his love since I was a little girl, wanting to do something so special that he would be proud of me. But it was like nothing I did was ever enough. I would never get what I wanted from him. Both men were gone from my life so I had to continue to put on my big girl panties and keep it moving.

2017 wasn't all bad. There were a lot of firsts. I did my first Spartan race. I won my first best actress award for the short film *Stain of Strife: Sins of the Family*. I got my motorcycle license and I bought my first motorcycle. I got my mastectomy tattoo. You have to remember the good because that will always outweigh the bad. It's what really matters because life stops for no one!

Note to self: You can't control how other people receive your energy. Anything you say or do gets filtered through the lens of whatever personal stuff they are going through at any given moment, which is not about you. Just keep doing YOU with as much integrity and love as possible.

As you have read, life is really good at throwing you for a loop or two or even three. I have been single for years. I stopped dating athletes and started dating blue collar types but things still aren't working out for me. They're too young, too controlling, drink too much, smoke too much weed, still looking for themselves, or not over an ex. My patterns have changed over the years but I still seem to attract or fall for the wrong guy. I have had four relationships in my life that have had a big impact on my development over the years:

- My first boyfriend, Reggie the Sailor, was eight years older than me. He was a friend of my brother-in-law.
- My ex-husband, Nate the football player.
- My first boyfriend after not dating athletes anymore – Derryl, the IT guy going into my late 30s.
- And William, the Marine, my long distance relationship whom I met online and thought was going to be my husband.

After years of saying I'm not desperate enough yet to have to use online dating, there I was making a profile. I had gotten online to start dating since my days of going to the club were over. I don't do much of anything but go to work, go to my acting classes, work on my projects, and go home. I started saying my boyfriend was my acting career. I really didn't want to date an actor because the community wasn't that big in Atlanta so I got on Match. Then I got on eHarmony with not much luck with either. I had two weeks left on my membership so I opened my account to the world. I heard from guys in Kentucky, North Carolina, and even Australia. I ended up connecting with William in Jacksonville, North Carolina.

I know I told myself I would never date a guy in the military again or one out of state, but I felt I was in a different place in my life. I was really ready for the right guy. I mean, at my age you know what you want and need for a healthy, thriving relationship. I still love my own space. I have been taking care of myself for so long but I will share it with the right one. He was getting ready to retire in four years so he would be land bound. We could live anywhere. I was a flight attendant with only an hour flight from Jacksonville. If it worked out, we would come up with a plan to live in the same city. That relationship lasted almost two years. I didn't date for a long time after that. My heart was broken. I thought he was the one.

After a year, he wanted me in North Carolina more but my life was in Atlanta. I had my acting career that he would say was just a hobby, asking how much longer I was going to do it. He pretty much wanted me to give up my passion for acting, retire from being a flight attendant and find a new career. He wanted me to change and adjust to his life. He wouldn't come out and exactly say that but it was implied and I thought I would be happy. However, without a proposal, I wasn't moving and he wasn't ready for that. We finally broke up at the end of July 2017. I have been single since then. I have dated a little and I got on a site called Bumble that lets the woman get in touch with the men first. I went on a couple dates but that didn't last very long. The last guy I dated was just trying to move so fast. He was a nice guy. His birthday was the same as my ex-

FREE ME 2 BE ME

boyfriend's and some of his mannerisms were the same. He took me to a Chris Brown concert and then I had to call it off. I mean he wasn't even my boyfriend. I barely kissed him. It just wasn't working for me. He wanted me to give him some more time to get to know him but I couldn't because the chemistry just wasn't there. I didn't even want to kiss him passionately. I would just give him a peck and he would say I kissed him like his grandma. I guess that should have been a big clue for him, but it wasn't. After that, I deleted all my online sites so if I meet someone, it will be the good old fashion way. Will I ever find a man who can put up with me? I know I can be a lot but I also know that I'm a great catch if the right guy can hook me. I sure hope I can write that chapter soon. Never underestimate a black woman born in August... a lot of sunshine mixed with a little hurricane.

1. Do you have any regrets in life? What is your biggest regret?

_____
_____
_____

2. What is your longest lasting relationship and with whom?

_____
_____
_____

3. What's your favorite vacation trip?

_____
_____
_____

4. What is on your bucket list for your next vacation?
_____
_____

5. Are YOU enough?
_____
_____
_____

> *"Opportunities don't just happen; you have to create them. Turn on the light and get to work. It's all in your attitude, so believe in yourself and know you can do it. I will get there, kicking and screaming and fighting all the way to the top. I will not be denied because I know that I'm enough!"*

CHAPTER TEN

LOOK AT ME NOW

Tattoo: A permanent design made on the skin with needles and ink, rhythmic tapping sound

ERIKA WEATHERS

I just celebrated 13 years being cancer free. My anniversary was June 3, 2021. I know that I am very blessed and I thank the Lord every day, but I still have insecurities and yes, that is my issue. When I first went through my reconstruction, they rebuilt my nipple, and tattooed my areola. It looked pretty good. You could still see a little of the scar but I was pretty happy with it and the skin was still supple. The second time, I didn't want to go that route. I still had some of the tattoo from the areola but the scar from the cut was more pronounced and a little darker because of the radiation, which was not very attractive.

I had been watching some tattoo shows on TV and saw an episode of a lady getting her breast tattooed so she could cover her scar. It was beautiful, so I started doing some research to find someone who could do one for me. I had also inquired about a 3D tattoo that was just a tattoo of a nipple. It had three dimensions and really looked like a nipple. It covered the scar pretty good but more of the scar then I wanted would still show. That would cost about $600 and insurance wouldn't cover it. The mastectomy tattoo could cost up to $1,000, depending on the artist. I found a website where artists were giving back and doing mastectomy tattoos for free, but I was about a year late.

I continued looking and found another lady, emailed her but I never heard back from her. When she finally responded, I had already found Jeff. It's so funny how the universe works with the power of positive thinking. I found an article about Jeff in the Montreal Gazette. He was offering free tattoos for breast cancer survivors. He was doing one lady a month. This was his way to give back instead of sending money. I loved it! I emailed him to find out if he was still taking new survivors. He said he was pretty booked for the year but since I only needed one breast done, he could squeeze me in. The only problem was that Jeff's studio was in Montreal, Canada. I mean it wasn't a major problem because I am a flight attendant but it would have been easier if it was in the states. Coincidentally, I had a trip scheduled to Montreal that next week. I made an appointment to meet Jeff and have a consultation about what I wanted.

I rented a car and met Jeff Wiens at his studio called Expressions. It was not far from my hotel, probably 20-30 minutes at the most. It was a straight shot after the turn-a-bout. I let him see my breast. He took some pictures and I told him what I was thinking about getting. I looked through some of his books to see his work and he also told me that he had worked on Angelina Jolie. I love her! She had both of her boobs removed, but he worked on her before all that.

I told him that I wanted to get some cherry blossoms with the tree bark and some butterflies and maybe some words. The meaning of the Japanese cherry blossom tattoo is both a feminine and fleeting reminder to live a life of beauty and to be present in the moment for that is all we have so seize it! Also to remember that nothing lasts forever, so appreciate the good stuff while it's in bloom. I love that it's also a symbol of Japanese warriors called samurai. The samurai serves to protect beauty and to preserve fine, delicate ways of life. They value beauty. They are more than just fierce warriors. Warriors are fearless and strong. The cherry tree is strong and hard but the blossoms are sweet and delicate. The butterfly represents endurance, change, hope and life. So, this is how I came up with the tattoo. All of those words encompass who I am! I made my appointment for Sep. 20, so in August I had to find a trip that had a long overnight and hoped and prayed that everything ran like clockwork.

I bid for that trip and everything went as planned. I told my crew what I was doing and my captain was like, "Are you sure you can get a tattoo on your overnight?" I was like, "Ahhh! Oh shit!" Well, it was too late because my appointment was the next morning. I went to the airport, grabbed breakfast, got my car rental and went to my appointment. Jeff sketched out what he was going to do, found some butterflies and we got started about 11 a.m. I made a live video of the before and after. I hadn't had a tattoo in a long time but I remember it didn't hurt too much. My pain threshold isn't too bad and with the numbness in some areas on my breast already it wasn't bad at all. It kind of felt good and I want to get another tattoo very soon. Crazy, huh? Pain and Pleasure...

Jeff bandaged me up, told me to keep it clean and put coconut oil on it so that it would heal. I made it back to the airport, changed into my uniform, went through customs and worked my flight back to the USA. It was so crazy how everything worked out perfectly. It was just meant to be.

When I got to the hotel that night, I took the bandage off because it had been on for too many hours. We didn't get to the hotel until about 9 p.m., so it needed to breathe. I cleaned it and put some coconut oil on it. I tried to sleep on my back with my boob uncovered, hoping I wouldn't get any color from the tattoo on the bed. I didn't have a good night's sleep that night but I didn't mess up the bed or my tat. It healed really nicely. I was so happy with it. It's so beautiful. I can't wait to do my photo shoot and show the world.

My tattoo is totally healed and it looks great. My doctor really liked it and was surprised that the scar took well to the ink. It's

FREE ME 2 BE ME

amazing how much more confident I am when taking my shirt off and I look at myself. I don't try to hide anymore. I am so proud of the way I look. It's not perfection, but I am so happy with my end result. If I do need another implant, it can be cut on the bottom of my breast and replaced.

I celebrated my 10 years of being cancer free on June 3, 2018. I had brunch with my family and friends. I got in trouble with a couple of my girlfriends who lived out of state for not inviting them. Even if they couldn't make it, I still should have invited them. Note to self: Don't forget to invite all my family and friends.

I had my event at one of my favorite spots in Midtown called Apres Diem. The room in the back is set up with couches and chairs. It's got an artsy flair to it that I like but the air conditioning wasn't working too great that day. Nonetheless, everyone survived. I had a really good turnout of about 20 people, from people coming early to some showing up later. The flow was great so I could spend some time with everyone. Another reason I love this spot is that everyone doesn't have to be there on time. I tried to get up and say thank you to everyone for coming and for always supporting me but I could hardly get anything out before crying. And, the cry was the ugly cry with very little words, all mixed together, trying to come out of my mouth to form a sentence. So, my cousin Doc had to come up and save me. He said some nice words and I just hugged and threw kisses to everyone. I hate when I can't control my emotions, especially as I keep getting older. I cry watching television shows, movies, commercials... Yes, commercials. I'm just an emotional creature who can't keep it together sometimes. I need to learn to use it in my acting auditions, how to turn it on and definitely when I need to turn it off.

The very next weekend, I was out at the pool with my niece and great nephew. The pool was pretty crowded and we had to sit on the other side from where we usually sat. There were tons of kids like someone went to the daycare, picked up some kids and dropped them all off but with only a couple adults supervising them. There were too many to be able to watch them all. Plus, we didn't have a lifeguard. I noticed that it looked like a kid was still under water for a long time. You know these kids like to try and hold their breath forever, but this was a little too long. We had one of the guys jump in and pull him out. He was drowning. A lady started CPR but it wasn't working so she stopped. I was like, "You can't just stop." So I started compressions and rescue breaths. Everything had gone quiet around me. People were calling 911. My niece and nephew were watching me. My flight attendant training had kicked in. It was like when I would practice on Bob the mannequin. In CPR training, we were taught 30 compressions and then 2 rescue breaths so that's what I was doing. I was counting 30 out loud then giving 2 breaths.

Water started coming out of his mouth but he was still unconscious. A guy wanted to help so I continued with the compressions and he did the rescue breathing. The boy finally came back to us. He was lifeless when I started on him. His eyes rolled back in his head and then he jumped up and was running around. I tried to get him to slow down and calm down. His family picked him up and brought him down to the ambulance. As quickly as it happened, it was over and the boy was gone. I didn't even get to find out what his name was, just that he was ok. He was probably 8 years old, the same age as my nephew. It was so surreal. I couldn't imagine how I would have felt if we lost him. I just kept at it hoping and praying he would wake back up and he did.

That day was one of my many "AHA!" moments. I was supposed to be there that day. At that time, I was saved so that I could save that little boy. It was emotional. I left the pool area and went and jumped on my motorcycle and went for a ride. My ex-boyfriend had just bought my motorcycle up from Jacksonville that April. I needed to feel the wind in my face. I needed to scream out loud and thank the Lord for helping me save that boy. I needed to be alone to just process what had just happened. It probably wasn't the greatest idea to jump on my bike when my mind was all over the place, but I returned home safely and sound. Remember everything happens for a reason. Our footsteps have already been mapped out, so continue to walk your path and pay attention.

I'm hoping to be able to display my tattoo in a coffee table book. I'm going to help get it together along with a few other projects to bring more exposure. The projects will reveal what happens to our bodies and the daily grind living with being cancer free, and how the chance of it coming back and becoming metastasis being pretty high, especially in the black community. We must learn how to live cleaner lives, watch what products we use and put into our bodies, eat healthier, minimize pesticides and carcinogen, and make fitness a daily practice in our lives. This should be done even if it's just 10 to 15 minutes a day because we have to do a better job of taking care of ourselves.

I have always been competitive; who doesn't like to win. But you must train to be the best. I set a lot of goals for myself after losing my job and I accomplished most of them in a short amount of time. When you put your mind, body and soul into anything and work hard, it can be done. I'm so proud of myself! I may be by myself and a little lonely having been isolated in the house because of COVID-19. But taking that time to continue to work on myself was very refreshing and so eye opening. I will continue to live every day to its fullest because I know how blessed I am to be here! Looking back on my life and retracing the steps that got me here, I can see decisions that I made. Some were just morphed into being, and some I had no choice but to take a leap to see where it would take me.

Overall, I think I'm a well-rounded individual with a good head on my shoulders and a heart of gold. Yes, I have made plenty of mistakes, learned from some, and repeated many, but God has a plan for me and it will be known soon! Yes, say it again! It will be known soon. Every mistake you make, God can make it a miracle. He can clean it up. I'm done. I'm bigger than my mistakes. It's my time! I don't have time for haters. I don't have time to waste worrying about foolishness. No time! I am more than just a pretty face. I have to listen and be obedient to God. Yes! Amen! Thank you Lord!

1. Do you embrace your flaws?
_____
_____
_____

2. Do you have tattoos?
_____
_____
_____

FREE ME 2 BE ME

3. What brings a smile to your face?

_____
_____
_____

4. What is the nicest thing that you have ever done for someone else?

_____
_____
_____

5. When was the last time you celebrated yourself?

_____
_____
_____

> *"Beauty is really just skin deep. We all lose it at some point. Will you still be shining when it's gone? Will your true beauty still come through? Remember, it's more important to have inner beauty that never goes away. It keeps that outer beauty around a whole lot longer. Keep Shining!"*

ERIKA WEATHERS

I AM ERIKA WEATHERS

Remember... don't sweat the really small stuff because tomorrow is never promised... So get out there and LIVE! These are the words I LIVE by. LIVE is in all caps because that's how I believe everyone should approach life - full of energy, enthusiasm, and always with a big exclamation point!

For as long as I can remember, I've craved adventure. When I was a little girl, I dreamed of being a cruise director on a giant boat, like Julie on the famous TV show, "The Love Boat", from the 80's. I grew up and became a flight attendant, so I didn't stray too far from that original dream. I've been flying for over 20 years now, but just recently furloughed due to the pandemic. I loved the flexible schedule it afforded me, as well as the extensive travel opportunities and the variety of people I get to meet and interact with on a daily basis. Health and wellness are a big part of my life, too. I am proud to say I'm a two-time breast cancer survivor. Later this year, I will celebrate my 13th year anniversary on June 3rd of being cancer free. The challenges I've faced have taught me that everyone has the power to take control of their own health, both physical and mental. Fitness is a big part of my life and I love spending time at the gym, working out and getting stronger. I also believe a strong mind and positive attitude are key components of success, and believing in yourself is just as necessary as working hard when it comes to achieving your dreams. For me, those dreams include going back to school to earn my second AA degree this time in criminal justice, training to be a motivational speaker, becoming a notary, a real estate agent and continuing to pursue my acting career. Life is a wonderful adventure and I plan to spend it learning and growing... and helping others do the same along the way.

FREE ME 2 BE ME

BY HIS STRIPES I AM...

I AM FORGIVEN FOR MY SINS

I AM HEALED

I AM THRIVING

I AM LOVED

I AM STRONGER

I AM RIGHTEOUS

I AM RESTORED

I AM RENEWED

I AM EDUCATED

I AM A SURVIVOR

I AM A WARRIOR

VICTORIOUS

Value: To be worthy or rate highly, cherish, consider precious, the importance or usefulness of something. Standards of behavior

Insecure: Not firmly fixed or attached, lacking confidence, anxious

Cancer: a malignant tumor of potentially unlimited growth that expands locally by invasion and systemically by metastasis.

Tattoo: A permanent design made on the skin with needles and ink, rhythmic tapping sound

Opinion: A personal view not necessarily based on fact or knowledge, the belief, judgement, impression or conviction of people in general.

Reassure: Put someone's mind at rest, encourage, cheer up, restore confidence

Identity: The distinguishing character or personality of an individual, specification, self

Obsession: a persistent disturbing preoccupation with an often unreasonable idea or feeling. Infatuation, fetish, fixation, passion

Use: The privilege or benefit of using something or someone, exploit unfairly, the power of control

Sex: Sexually motivated phenomena or behavior, copulation, fornication

ABOUT THE AUTHOR

Erika Weathers is a two-time Breast Cancer Survivor born in Middletown New York now residing in Atlanta Georgia since 1996. She is a daughter, sister, aunt, and advocate. She is single with no kids and has an Associate Degree in Art. For the last 20+ years she has been a Flight Attendant. She is a Licensed Real Estate Agent, a Notary, Secretary of the Neighborhood Planning Unit M (NPU-M) Public Safety for the City of Atlanta as well as an aspiring Actress, Biker Chick and first-time Author. She enjoys staying active & fit and her favorite place is the beach.

ERIKA WEATHERS

Made in the USA
Columbia, SC
09 October 2021